Braids

Easy Step-by-Step Hairstyles

Hair Designer
Mary Beth Janssen-Fleischman

Contributing Writer
Judy Rambert

D0956626

Publications International, Ltd.

CONTENTS

Louis Weber, C.E.O.
Publications International, Ltd.
7373 North Cicero Avenue
Lincolnwood, Illinois 60646

Permission is never granted for commercial purposes.

Manufactured in Austria

8 7 6 5 4 3 2 1

Hair Designer **Mary Beth Janssen-Fleischman** is International Artistic Director for Pivot Point Beauty School.

Contributing Writer **Judy Rambert** is Vice President of Education for Pivot Point Beauty School.

Photographers: Irena Lukasiewicz, David Puffer
Photography Assistant: Ed Ernst

Hair Stylist: Mary Beth Janssen-Fleishman
Assistant Stylist: Barbara Kauth
Makeup Artist: Karen Lynn

Models:
Royal Model Management: Pamela Berk, Laura Truxler, Stephanie Loyola, Laurie White, Raheda Shurn, Amanda Sassano, Barb Horn, Lisa Myles; **The Models Workshop Studio:** Suzanne Favors; Donna Wieczorkowski.

INTRODUCTION

Even with designer clothing, perfectly applied makeup, and fine jewelry, no look is really complete without a distinctive hairstyle to top it off. Unique and striking hair designs have been a part of the fashion world throughout history, and braiding has consistently been one of the most effective ways to design individual styles. By combining various braid techniques and applying them in different ways, you can create a whole range of statements, from sophisticated and elegant to carefree and casual. You can develop styles that work well for the young or old, that are suitable for any occasion, that match a particular mood or outfit, or that are just plain fun to do. You can give yourself a whole new look any time you want, and perhaps best of all, you can change the way you look tomorrow if you decide you don't like it.

Once you master some of the basic techniques in this book, you can create many of your own designs at home. As in any art form, the more you practice, the better you become. The designs featured in this book have been created by a very skilled professional, so don't be discouraged if your first results are not an exact duplicate. Our intent is to show you some classic techniques that you can use on yourself, your friends, or your family between professional salon visits. So have some fun, experiment with the designs we feature, and create some of your own.

A note about the instructions in this book: To avoid confusion, we have used the terms "left" and "right" to refer to the *reader's* left and right.

TECHNIQUES

BRAIDS

Two basic techniques create three-strand braided designs. One is **overbraiding**, and the other is **underbraiding**. In overbraiding, the outside strands are crossed over the center strand. In underbraiding, the outside strands are crossed under the center strand. Braids created with an overbraid technique have also been called English braids; those with an underbraid technique have been called Dutch braids. The choice between overbraiding or underbraiding depends upon your personal preference and which technique is more comfortable for you to perform.

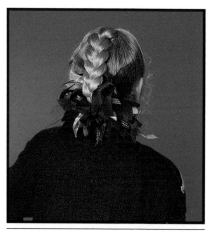

Overbraid

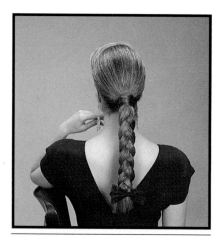

Underbraid

When these two techniques are performed on free-hanging ponytails, there is only a slight difference in the braided pattern. The visible difference occurs when these techniques are combined with the addition of new sections of hair gathered from the scalp and added to the outside strands while you continue to braid. Overbraiding with added sections, which is also known as a French braid, produces a flat or **inverted braid** pattern. When you incorporate new sections of hair while underbraiding, the result will be a raised or **projected braid**. This technique creates corn-row designs, along with many other styles.

We have also incorporated a **four-strand round braid** into some of these designs. This technique makes an unusual-looking chainlike braid, and it's not difficult to master. The outside strands are brought under two strands and back over one.

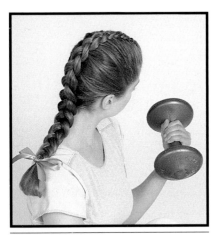

Projected Underbraid

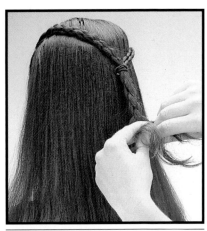

4-Strand Round Braid

TWO-STRAND OVERLAP

This technique features only two strands, which are alternately crossed from one side to the other side. The technique can be performed on the free ends of a ponytail or along the scalp with new sections added. The result is a beautiful herringbone pattern, which has also been called a fish tail.

TWISTS

The other technique featured in the book is twisting. Individual strands can be twisted independently, or two strands can be twisted together. The resulting pattern resembles a rope. This technique can be performed on the free ends of a ponytail, or the twist can be combined with new additions picked up along the hairline that are incorporated into the twist.

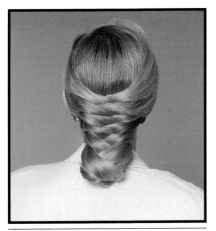

Two-Strand Overlap

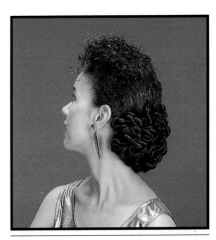

Twist

HAIR WRAPPING

For a more dressed look, cover the band securing the ponytail with hair.

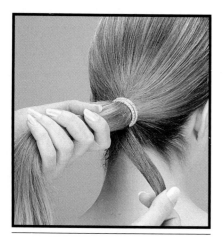

1. Select a small portion of hair from underneath the ponytail.

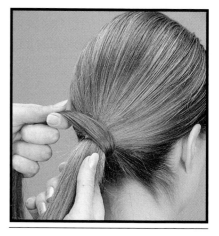

2. Wrap the hair around the base of the ponytail to hide the covered band.

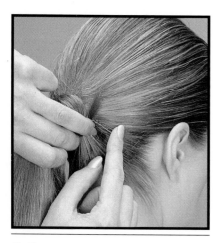

3. Fasten the wrap by inserting a hairpin.

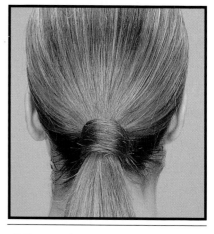

4. The result is a simple, yet beautiful, complement to any design.

SPIRAL WRAPPING

By wrapping a cord or ribbon in a spiral fashion around the braid ends, you can cover a band or even eliminate it entirely.

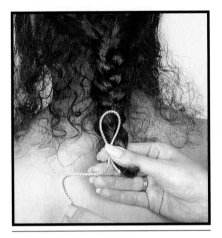

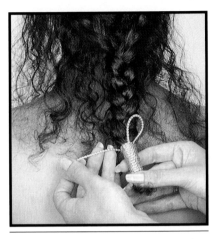

1. Select a long cord, at least ten or twelve inches in length. Loop one end and hold it next to the ends of the hair.

2. Wrap the loose end around the hair from the bottom upward.

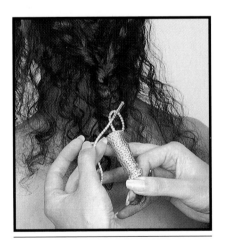

3. When you get toward the top and enough of the loop is still showing, insert the end of the cord through the loop.

(continued)

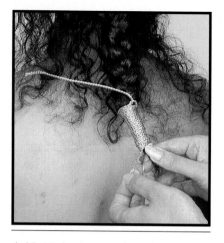

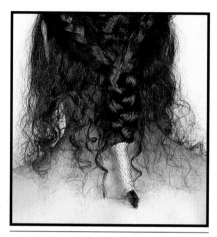

4. Hold the hair end as shown and pull slowly on the bottom end of the cord until the loop disappears inside the wrapped area. Clip off the extra cord ends on the top and bottom.

5. The result looks more difficult than it really is. Vary the effect by using different types of cord or ribbon to complement your wardrobe or reflect the mood of the finished design.

BEADED FINISH

When selecting beads, consider their color and weight and the amount of light they reflect. Glass beads reflect the most light; plastic and wood weigh the least. Avoid putting heavy beads on fragile hair.

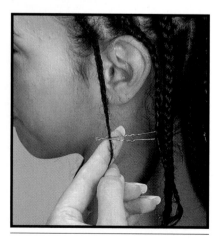

1. Begin by squeezing the closed end of a hairpin to make it smaller. Then place the end of the braid between the open ends of the hairpin.

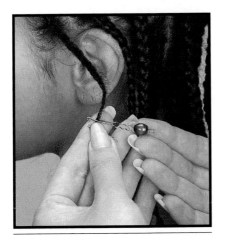

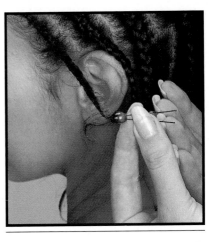

2. Insert both prongs of the hairpin through the hole in the bead.

3. Thread the bead onto the braid by pulling the pin through the bead.

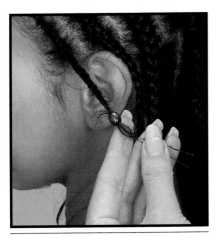

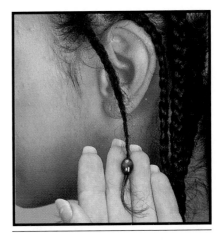

4. Move the bead along the length of the braid, positioning it where it looks best.

5. The bead should fit snugly, so if the opening is too large, you may need either to move the bead higher up the braid or choose another bead.

PRODUCTS

POMADE

Use a pomade to remove static, control flyaway ends, and add a glossy sheen to either straight or curly hair. Pomade should be used sparingly, though. Apply a very small amount to one hand and liquefy it between your palms. Then run your hands through the hair before braiding or use it for small touch-ups afterward.

GEL

Gel will control hair lengths too, but it produces more of a wet effect than pomade does. You can apply gel to all of the hair before you braid, or, when you want a clean, off-the-face effect, you can apply it to the perimeter hairline where lengths tend to be shorter. Gel can also be used after a braid is finished to smooth down loose or uncontrolled hairs. Apply it to your fingertip or to the end of a hairpin; then direct it on top of the stray hairs to encourage them back into the braided pattern.

HAIR SPRAY

Besides using hair spray to hold the finished design in place, try using it in spot areas as you work. Also, if you want to create a soft finish but need to control the hair, spray lightly into the palm of your hand and then smooth over the surface of the hair to control flyaway strands before you braid.

COATED BANDS

Ordinary rubber bands can place undue tension on the hair, which may cause hair breakage. Using a coated rubber band to secure ponytails and the ends of a braid will reduce the stress on the hair. This extra consideration will help keep your hair in better condition.

ACCESSORIES

Adding an ornament, barrette, ribbon, or any of the wide assortment of accessories available can finish your completed design. The selection is based on practical purposes—to keep ends secure—as well as decorative options. Both the occasion and your wardrobe should influence the type of accessory you select and the way that you work it into the hairstyle.

For business, simplicity is generally the key. For active sports, choose barrettes, grips, or ribbons that adhere with tension. For special occasions, pearls or silver and gold ornaments give extra elegance and sophistication. Don't forget a great standby—flowers, either fresh or silk. From large dahlias to smaller baby's breath, flowers pinned into the design can add a touch of romantic femininity.

Remember, not every design requires accessorizing; sometimes the pattern in the hair is enough. If you do choose ornamentation, make sure that it matches the feeling that you want to portray.

Your professional salon, as well as hobby craft stores, fabric stores, and millinery sections of departments stores, can all be resources for you to find the right accessory to add the final touch to your design.

SLEEK AND MODERN

FIGURE-EIGHT OVERBRAID

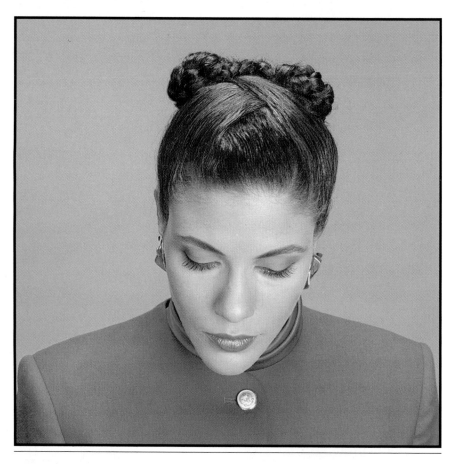

This classic look is suitable for either business or evening wear. The pattern at the top of the head is composed of two braids arranged like a figure eight. Here we've positioned the two braids so that the figure eight is horizontal, but you can also create a vertical design. The size and shape of the figure eight will depend upon how long the hair is and how far apart you place the ponytails before they are braided.

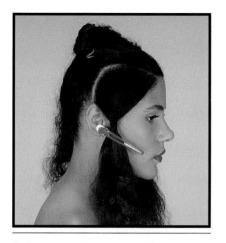

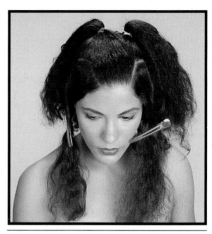

1. Section off an area of hair on each side of the head with curved partings and secure each section with a clip. Brush the remaining hair smooth and form it into two ponytails side by side at the top of the head.

2. Notice that the front hairline between the curved partings is included in the ponytails.

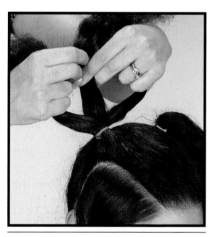

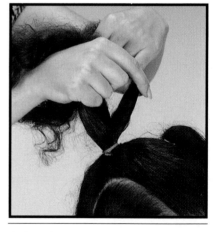

3. Braid each ponytail using the overbraid technique. Begin by dividing one of the ponytails into three equal-size strands.

4. Reach across to grasp the right strand with your thumb and forefinger.

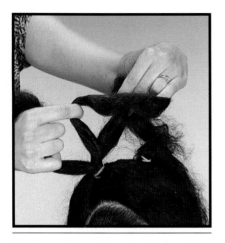

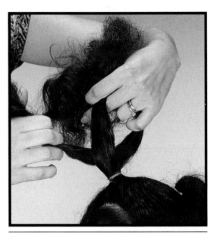

5. Cross this right strand over the center strand so that the right strand is now the center strand.

6. Reach across to the left side and grasp the left strand. Cross it over the center strand so that it is in the center position. Continue overbraiding down the length of the ponytail. Secure the ends with a coated band.

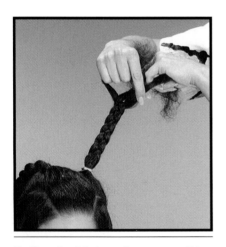

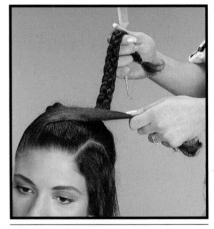

7. Overbraid the other ponytail in the same way. Secure the ends with a coated band.

8. Unclip the left side section and comb it smoothly upward, directing it over the top and around the braid on the right.

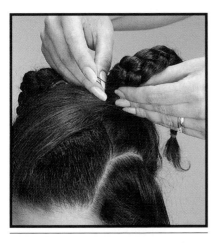

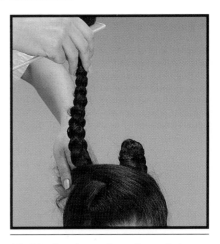

9. Curve the ends around the base of the braid and pin with hairpins to secure it.

10. Unclip the right side and direct it over the top of the head. Wrap the end around the base of the braid on the left and secure it with hairpins.

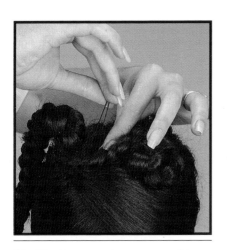

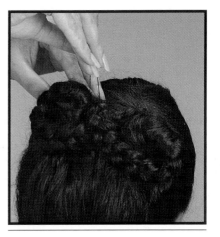

11. The figure eight is created last. Curve the right braid back to form a loop and then forward around the base of the braid on the opposite side. Pin the end of the right braid to the base of the opposite braid.

12. Repeat step 11 for the left braid. You can experiment by creating different shapes, depending on the length of the braids.

PATTERNED ELEGANCE

THREE-STRAND OVERBRAID WITH CROWN KNOT

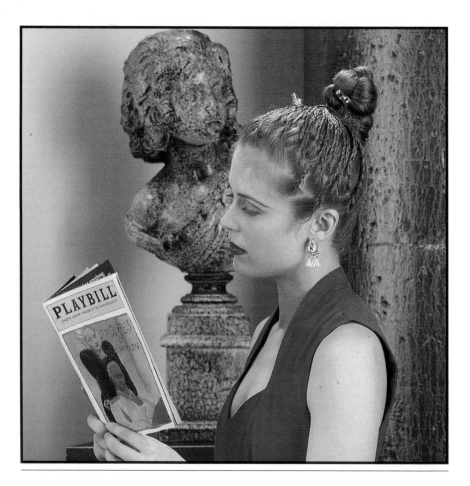

This imaginative design creates excitement with different three-strand braid sizes. A large braid forms the crown topknot, while delicate three-strand braids trace over the smooth, pulled-back hair to encircle the base of the topknot.

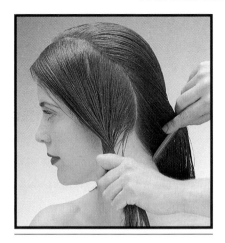

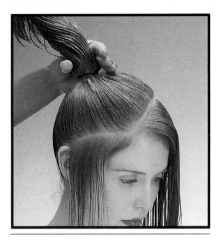

1. Begin with hair that is dampened and gelled. Part diagonally from the right front hairline area over the head to behind the left ear. Leave this hair hanging free for now.

2. Part a small diagonal section on the side above the right ear. Fasten the rest of the hair with a coated elastic band into a ponytail at the upper crown area. (Exclude hair from step 1.)

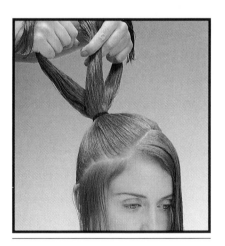

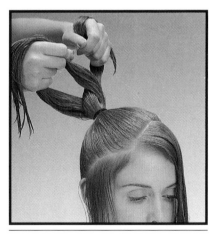

3. Divide this ponytail into three equal strands in preparation for the three-strand overbraid. Reach over with the left hand and, with index finger and thumb, grasp the outside right strand and cross it over the center strand.

4. Reach over with the right hand and, with index finger and thumb, grasp the left strand and cross it over the center strand. Repeat this crossover technique to the ends and fasten with a coated elastic band.

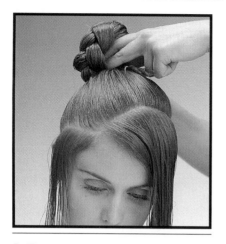

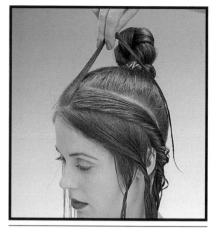

5. To create the topknot, place two fingers at the base of the braid. Wrap the braid clockwise around the fingers, working close to the head. Tuck the ends beneath the topknot and pin them in place.

6. Divide the free-hanging hair on the left side into three sections. Beginning in the top section near the front hairline, part a small subsection on an angle. Comb and direct this subsection back toward the topknot.

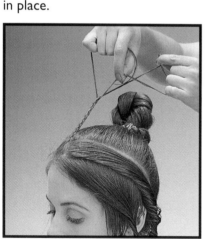

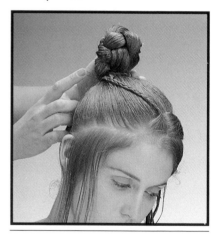

7. Divide the subsection into three equal strands and start a three-strand overbraid as described in steps 3 and 4.

8. Continue to the ends of the subsection and use the braid to encircle the ponytail base. Pin in place to secure.

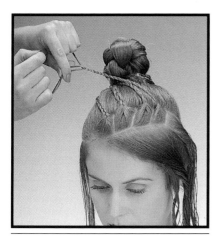

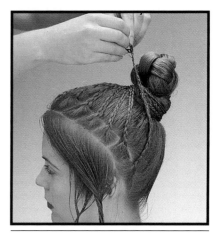

9. Continue making small braids within the section, working toward the area behind the ear. Maintain angled partings for each subsection. Encircle the ponytail's base with each braid. Pin in place.

10. When you reach the area behind the ear, direct the hair upward and toward the front of the knot as you braid. Encircle the topknot and pin in place.

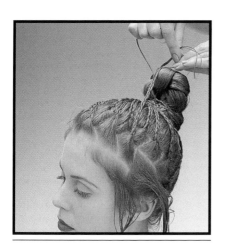

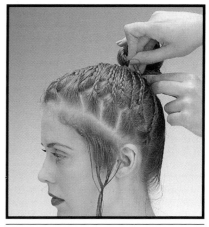

11. Continue into the next section. Reverse the parting angle and braid each subsection in this area up and toward the topknot.

12. Fasten each braid around the base of the knot with a hairpin.

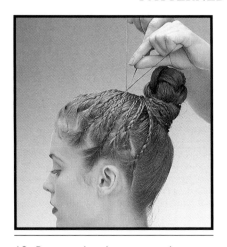 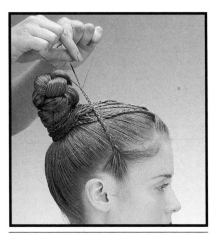

13. Repeat the three-strand overbraid technique in the final section. Reverse the parting angles for the subsections.

14. Create one or more decorative braid accents with the section on the right side, braiding up and toward the topknot.

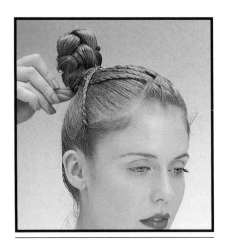 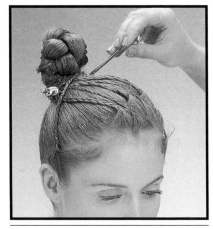

15. Encircle the base of the topknot with this braid and secure with a hairpin.

16. A decorative hair pick adds not only an ornamental effect, but also an extra measure of security to the topknot.

CHARMINGLY CHIC

DRAPED OVERBRAID

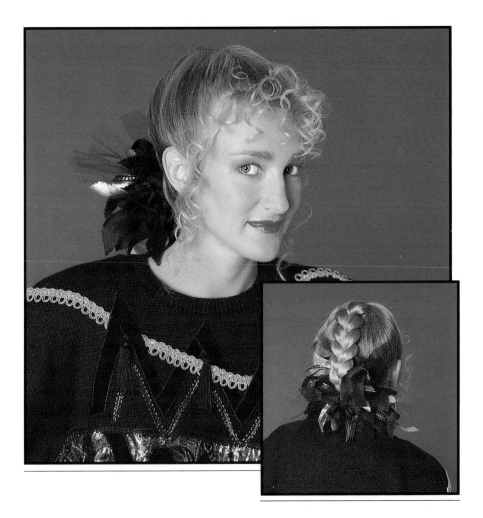

This design requires hair long enough to reach at least halfway down the back. The lengths are gathered at the top of the head and braided; the braid is then draped down the center back of the head. It's surprisingly easy to do on your own hair. We've braided the hair dry, which causes a slight drape in the hair around the face. If you braid the hair while it is wet, the hair will remain very close to the head.

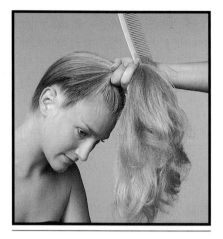

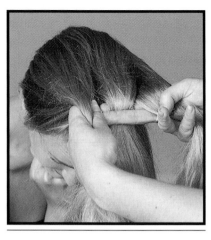

1. Comb all the hair smoothly upward to the top of the head. If necessary to control stray strands, mist the hairline with water or hair spray.

2. Divide the hair into three equal-size sections.

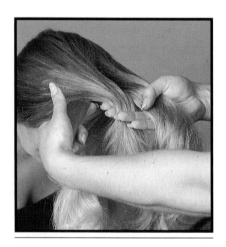

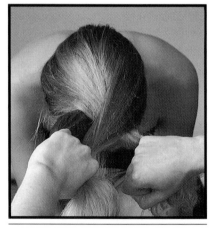

3. Cross the left strand over the center strand. The center strand moves to the left and the left strand now becomes the center strand.

4. Reach over and grasp the right strand. Direct it over the center strand. The right strand now becomes the center strand.

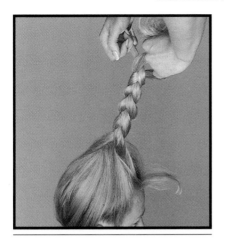

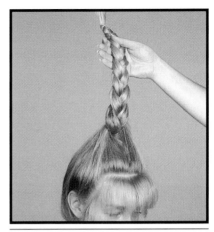

5. Repeat the procedure by continuing to cross the side strands over the center strands, alternating left and right. Keep the head bent down to make braiding easier.

6. Overbraid down the length of the hair and secure the ends with a band. Lift the braid straight upward, allowing shorter fringe lengths to fall down naturally. These lengths can be left straight or curled with a curling iron later.

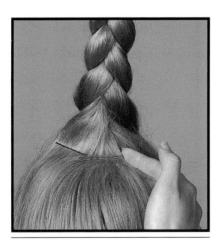

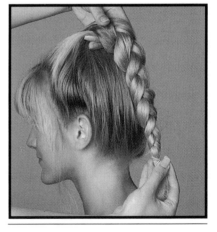

7. Pin behind the base of the braid with bobby pins to secure the hair upward.

8. Fold the braid over the pins and drape it down the center of the head.

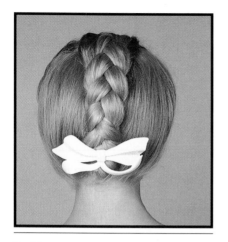

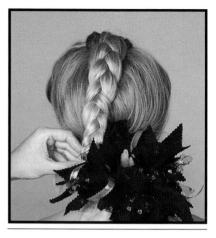

9. Choose ornamentation to match the occasion and the colors being worn. For a casual look, secure a barrette or small bow to the end of the braid.

10. For a more formal version, try an ornamental elastic holder. The hole in this ornament allows you to insert the end of the braid into the holder.

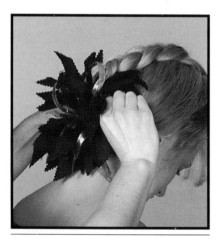

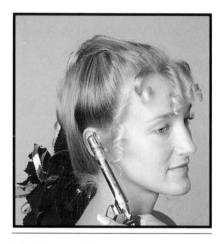

11. Secure the end of the hair with a bobby pin to position both the braid and the ornament. Pin around the ornament in several places.

12. Shorter fringe lengths around the face can be incorporated casually by releasing them and curling them with a curling iron for a soft finish.

CLASSIC BEAUTY

OVERBRAID CHIGNON

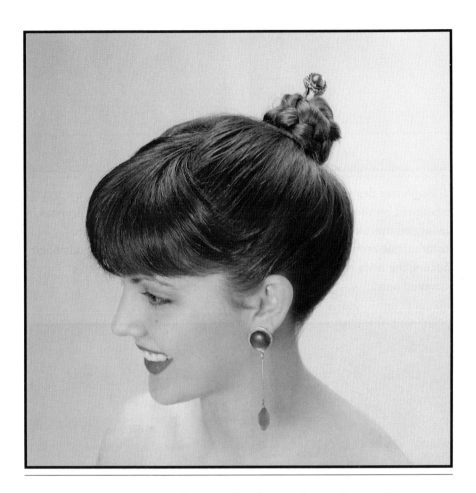

You can quickly transform a classic overbraid into a chignon. The main requirement for this design is a braided length that is long enough to turn a complete circle around the base of a ponytail and allow the ends to be tucked under. Vary the expression of this design by changing the location of the ponytail from the crown of the head to the nape—the back of the neck. If you have shorter lengths around the face, they can be left out of the ponytail and styled independently.

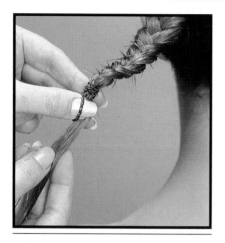

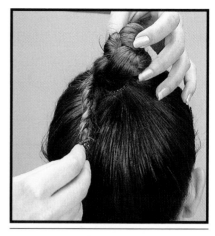

1. Begin this design by positioning a ponytail on the crown and then using the overbraiding technique to braid the remaining lengths. Secure the ends with a small covered band.

2. Wrap the finished braid, curving it around the base of the ponytail. The center will rise upward slightly. That's supposed to happen to achieve the shape of this chignon.

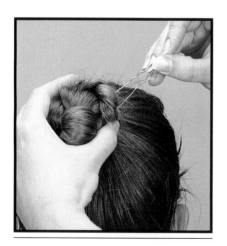

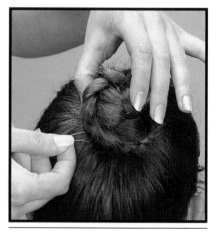

3. Cup one hand around the chignon, and then secure its position by inserting a large hairpin into the coil and the hair underneath it.

4. Tuck the ends under and secure them with small bobby pins. If the hair is very heavy, you may achieve a better hold with large pins or several small ones.

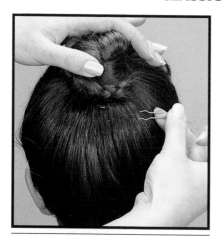 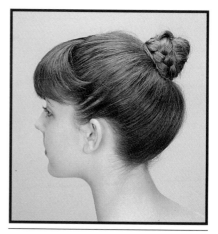

5. Balance the volume of the design by inserting a hairpin into any low areas and lifting the hair outward. Spray with hair spray to hold the new shape.

6. Shorter bang lengths were left out of the ponytail and styled smooth, but if your hair is longer at the front you can style it off the face and include it in the ponytail. Accessories and ornaments are optional on the finished design.

INGENUE

HALO OVERBRAID

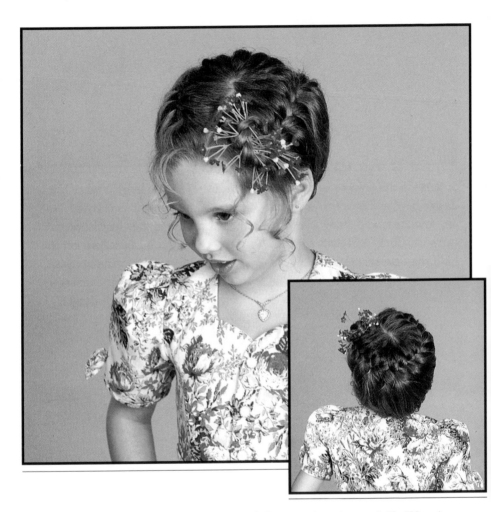

This braid is perfect for a special occasion in a girl's life. A few loose tendrils soften the area around the face, and you can incorporate dried flowers to customize the design by repeating wardrobe colors. Even distribution of the hair around the curve of the head is important. In this technique hair is picked up and added to the outside strands of the overbraid. This design can also be done on wet hair, which creates a more casual finish that lies closer to the head.

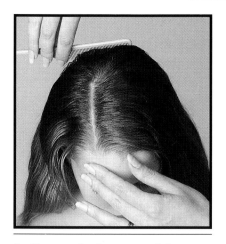

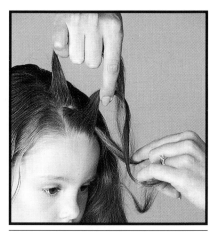

1. Choose the location of the braid. The location will determine how you distribute the hair. For this design, the hair was distributed off a short side part. Mist the hair lightly with water to control the hair before braiding.

2. Section a triangular area on the side of the part with the most hair. Subdivide it into three equal-size strands. Cross the right strand over the center strand so that the right strand is now in the center position.

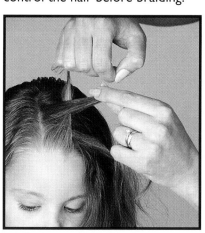

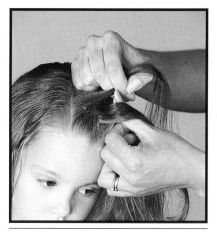

3. Grasp the left strand and cross it over the center strand so that the left strand moves into the center position. Keep your hands close to the head.

4. Release the right strand into the hair below. Pick up a new section of hair from the area between the hairline and the braid. Pick up the dropped strand with this new section.

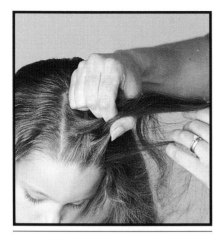

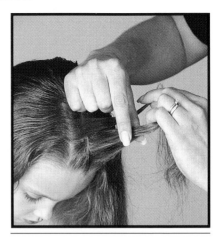

5. Drape the new section on your thumb. Run your hand down the length of the hair to clear the strand from the hair below.

6. Transfer the center strand and the new strand to the opposite hand. Grasp the new, combined strand with your thumb and forefinger.

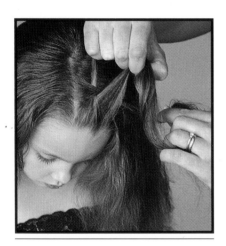

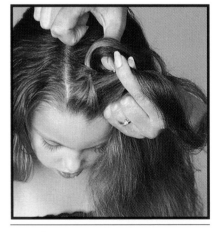

7. Cross the new strand over the center strand.

8. Now release the strand on the left into the hair below. Use your thumb to pick up a new section of hair from the area between the part and the braid. Pick up the dropped strand with the new section.

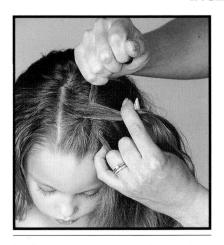

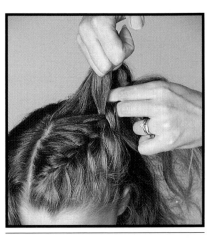

9. Cross this new strand over the center strand, and tighten up any slack in the strands.

10. Continue around the curve of the head, trying to pick up equal amounts of hair each time and maintaining symmetry. Mist the hair with water periodically to control stray strands. This is especially helpful if the hair is wavy.

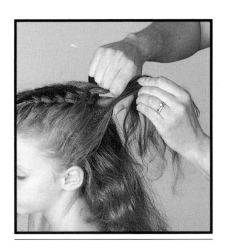

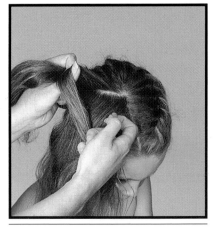

11. Direct the braid so that it curves around the back of the head. As you round the back, include all of the hair from the nape in the picked-up sections.

12. To pivot the pattern of picked-up sections around the end of the part, section triangular areas radiating from the end of the part.

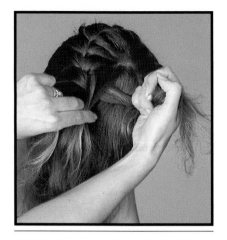

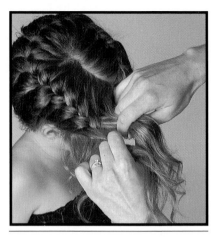

13. Continue overbraiding on the other side, keeping the braid high and balanced with the first side. Remember to keep your hands close to the head to maintain tension.

14. Continue the curve to form a braided circle on the top of the head.

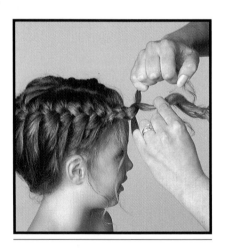

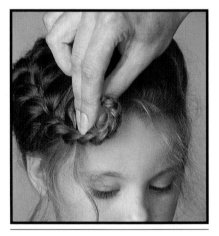

15. Once you have picked up all of the hair from the scalp, continue to overbraid the remaining loose hair.

16. Secure the ends with a coated elastic band and coil the free part of the braid into a tight circle.

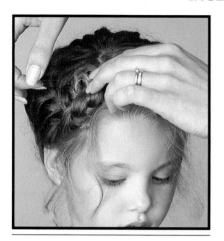 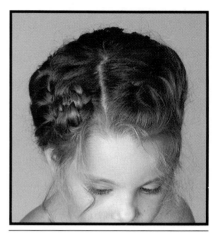

17. Pin the braid into position with hairpins.

18. An optional step is to release a few strands near the hairline to soften the line around the face. If you wish, you can curl the strands with a curling iron.

ELEGANT SIMPLICITY

UNDERBRAID

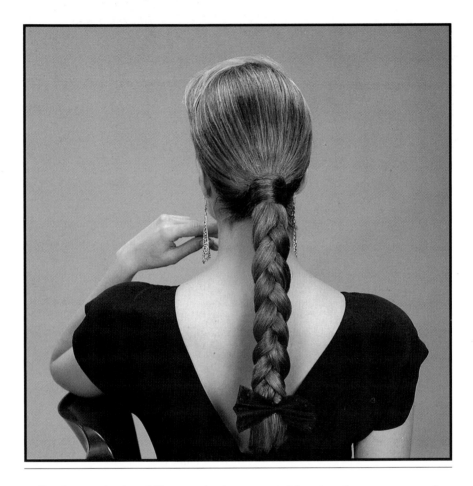

In the underbraiding technique, outside stands are crossed *under* the center strand. This produces a plump-looking braid that is also called a Dutch braid. Begin with a simple ponytail to learn the basics. When you are familiar with the pattern, experiment with it to create your own interpretations. Once mastered, this basic technique can be used alone or in combination with other techniques.

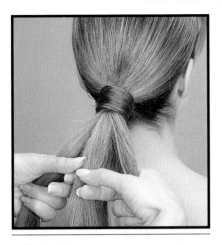

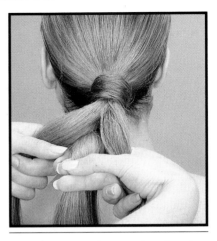

1. Begin by creating a ponytail where you would like the braid positioned. For this design we chose the lower nape. Divide the ponytail into three equal-size strands.

2. Direct the left strand under the center strand. The center strand moves to the left and the left strand becomes the center strand.

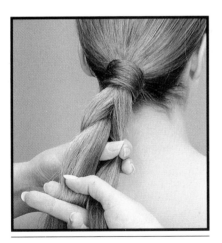

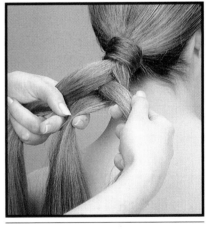

3. Reach under the center and grasp the right strand with your thumb and index finger.

4. Direct it under the center. The right strand now exchanges positions with the center strand.

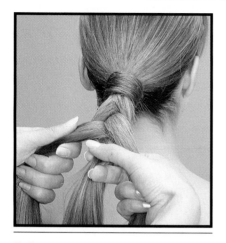

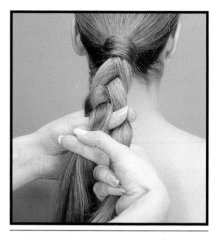

5. Repeat this basic pattern. Direct the left strand under the center strand.

6. Grasp the right strand with your thumb and index finger and direct it under the center.

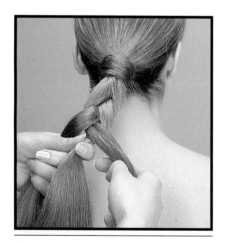

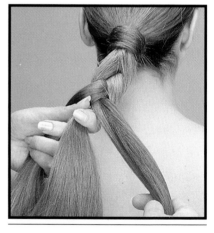

7. As you braid you will be holding two strands in one hand and one strand in the other hand, which will alternate. Your braids will be neater if you slide your hand down the length of the strands every so often to smooth stray hairs.

8. Smooth the side with one strand as you maintain tension on the other two strands with the other hand.

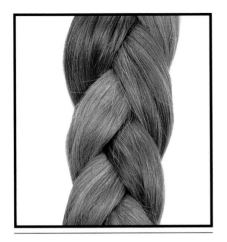

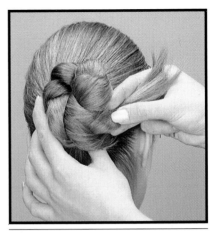

9. Continue underbraiding down the length of the strands. Finish the braid by securing the ends with a covered band or wrapping them with a cord or thread. This creates the basic style shown on page 36.

10. If your hair is long enough, you can create a chignon. Coil the braid around the base of the ponytail. Hold the braid against the head to keep it flat. Wrap the ends under the braid and tuck them into the center.

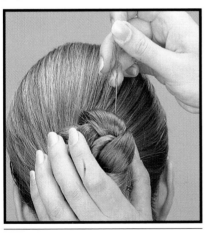

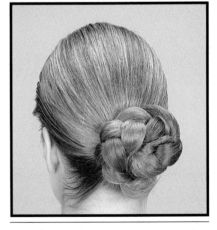

11. Hold the coil with one hand and insert a large hairpin into the chignon to hold it in position. Additional pins will be necessary to secure the chignon if your hair is heavy.

12. This design has a classical appeal and can be varied by changing the location of the chignon and by adding different ornamentation.

ACTIVE HAIR

PROJECTED UNDERBRAID

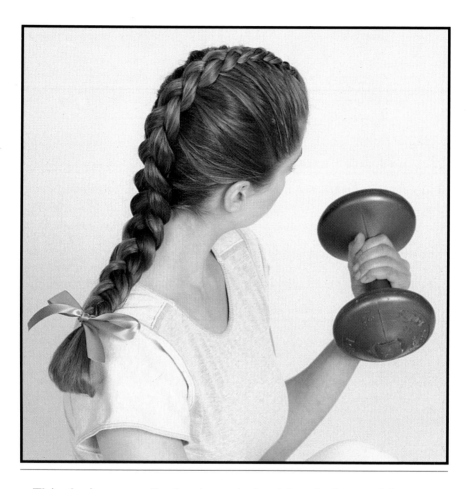

This design uses the basic underbraid technique with new sections of hair added in to the outside strands as you braid. The outside strands are always crossed under the center, which results in a braided pattern that projects upward. Adjust the size of the picked-up sections according to the intricacy of the pattern you would like to create. This version positions a single braid down the center from the front hairline to the nape. The same braid can be created from a side part or combined with several small braids positioned across the head.

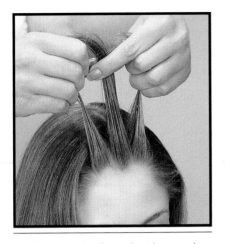

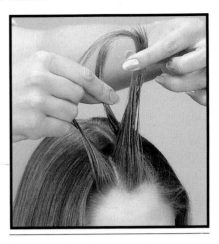

1. Begin at the front hairline and create a triangular section. Divide the section into three equal-size strands.

2. Cross the right strand under the center strand. The right strand now becomes the center strand, and the center strand becomes the right strand.

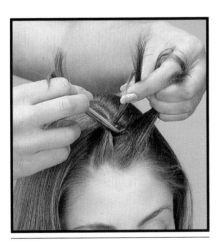

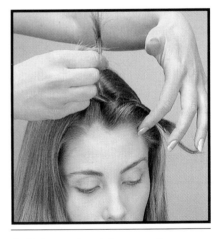

3. Now cross the left strand under the center strand. This positions the left strand in the center.

4. Release the right strand.

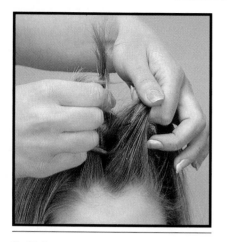

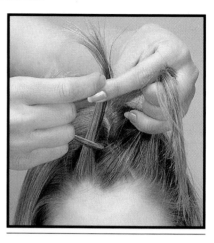

5. Pick up a new section of hair on the right side from the hairline to the center part. Include the right strand you have just dropped, creating a new, combined strand.

6. Shift the center strand to your right hand.

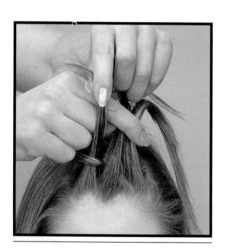

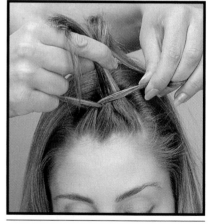

7. Extend your thumb and index finger to reach under to grasp the new, combined strand.

8. Direct the combined strand under the center and pull the strands taut.

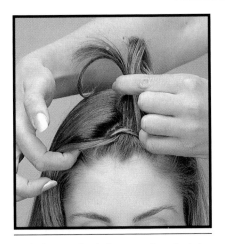

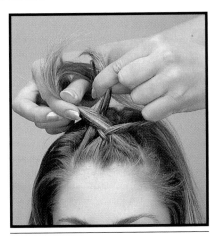

9. Release the left strand and pick up a new section of hair from the hairline to the top of the head.

10. Reach under with your thumb and index finger to grasp the combined strand and cross it under the center.

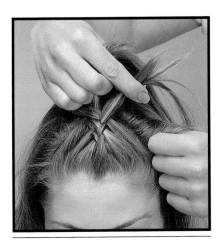

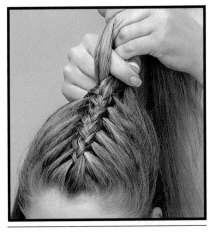

11. If you are braiding in shorter layers, you may have to hold the outside strands and direct the new sections upward toward them, rather than releasing the outside strand and picking it back up as you gather the new sections.

12. Pick up the new sections from the hairline to the top of the head and cross them under the center strand. Try to keep the size of the picked-up sections consistent.

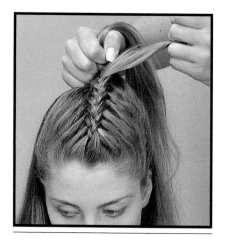

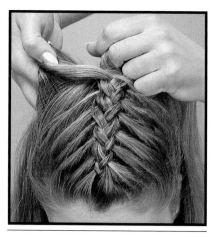

13. Slide your hand down the strands every so often to untangle and smooth the lengths.

14. Pick up new sections of hair from alternate sides.

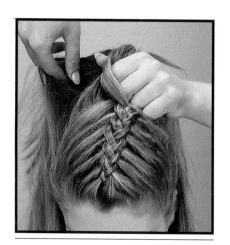

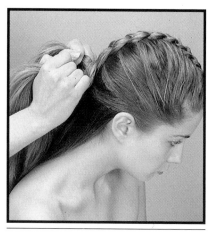

15. Clear away the rest of the hair as you hold the new addition with your thumb.

16. Stay close to the head and maintain tension.

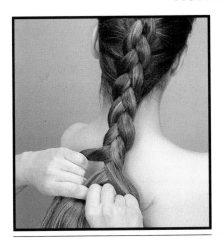 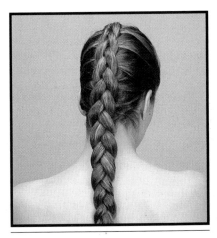

17. Once you have picked up the last sections of hair, continue with the basic underbraid pattern on the ends.

18. Secure the ends with a band and cover it decoratively, if you wish.

SOPHISTICATE

RIBBON UNDERBRAID

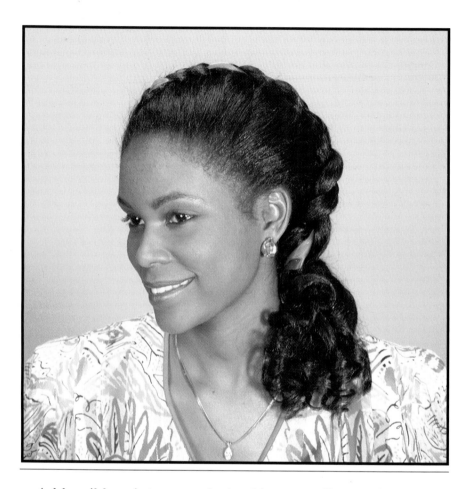

Add a ribbon into an underbraid to coordinate with your wardrobe. This asymmetrical underbraid travels from above the eye on one side up over the curve of the head to the opposite side behind the ear. The longer nape lengths are left loose to be gathered by the braid. Whether straight, wavy or curly, these ends are fanned out to add volume and fullness.

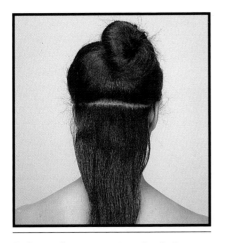

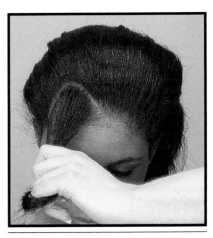

1. Begin by sectioning the hair to separate the area to be under-braided from the loose areas. This sectioning can vary depending upon the amount of hair you want to leave loose at the nape.

2. Select a triangular section slightly off center.

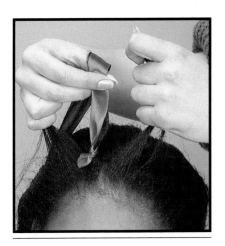

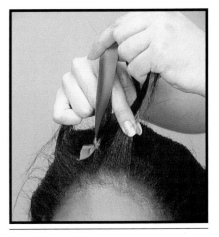

3. Divide this section into three strands and tie a ribbon to the center strand, draping it back. Trim the ends of the ribbon as needed. Various sizes and types of ribbon can be chosen to customize the design.

4. The ribbon will follow the path of the center strand. Cross the right strand under the center strand.

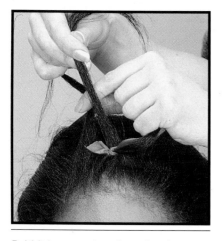

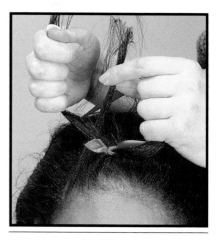

5. With your thumb and index finger, reach over and grasp the left strand.

6. Direct it under the center strand to the middle position.

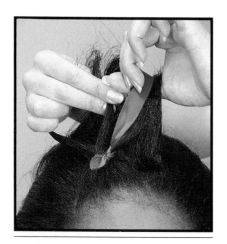

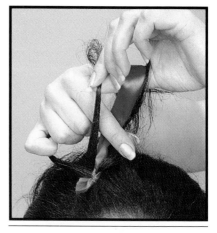

7. Comb through the scalp area to the center with your thumb, picking up the new section. Combine the new section with the outside strand and hook it over your thumb.

8. Your thumb and index finger are now free to grasp the center strand, allowing the opposite thumb and index finger to reach under and grasp the outside strand.

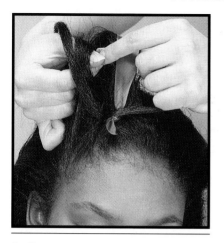

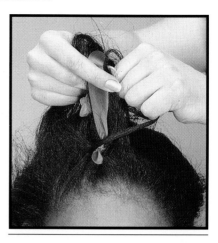

9. Continue this exchange, alternating from side to side.

10. Reach under with the opposite hand and grasp the left outside strand with your thumb and index finger, and cross the strand under to the center position.

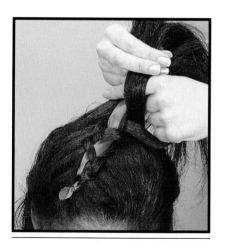

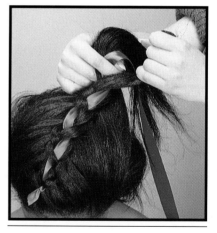

11. Continue braiding toward the back of the head. Maintain tension and work close to the head.

12. As you cross the outside strands under the center, try not to let the ribbon roll inside the braid. For the best effect, keep the ribbon visible and lying on top of the strand.

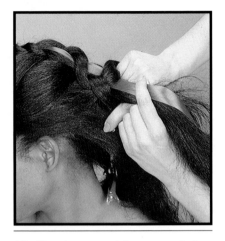

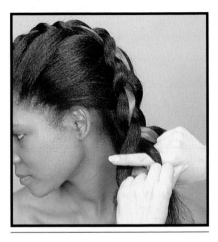

13. Continue to pick up new hair sections and add them to the outside strands before crossing under, until you reach the back area where the hair has been divided.

14. At this point, use the basic underbraiding technique through to the ends.

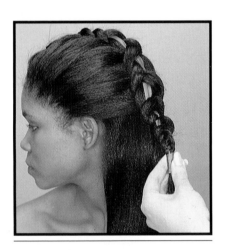

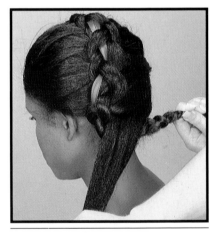

15. Encircle the ends with the ribbon, and tie it into a knot or pin it with a bobby pin.

16. Wrap this braid completely around the loose hair at the nape.

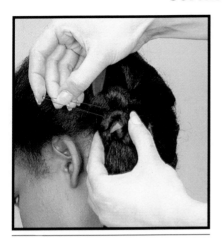

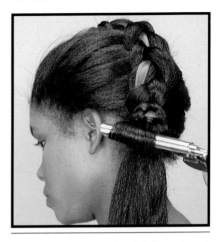

17. Pin in place securely with a hairpin and/or a bobby pin.

18. The ends may be left loose and straight or curled with a curling iron or hot rollers. The ribbon braid could easily be incorporated all the way to the ends, if you wish.

SPIRITED TEXTURE

PROJECTED UNDERBRAID WITH CENTER PART

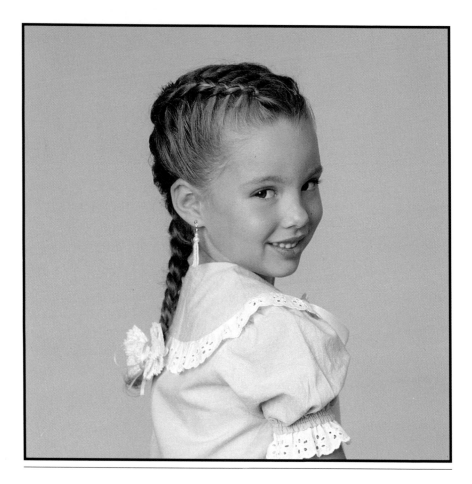

This style is a good choice either for a young girl or as an active style for a young woman. The two sides are underbraided, and the two underbraids are joined at the center back to produce a large underbraid that hangs free. The underbraids project from the head, creating an interesting graphic design.

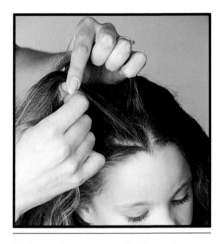

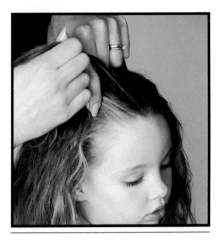

1. Begin by parting the hair down the center and combing each side smooth. Select a triangular section of hair from the front of one side and divide it into three equal-size strands.

2. Reach under and grasp the left strand.

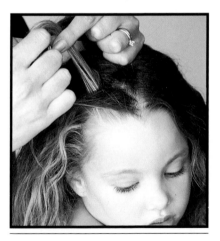

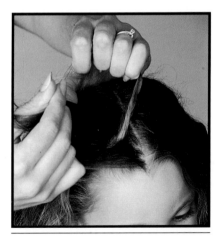

3. Cross the left strand under the center strand so that the left strand is now in the center position.

4. Reach under to grasp the right strand. Cross the right strand under the center strand so that the right strand is now in the center position.

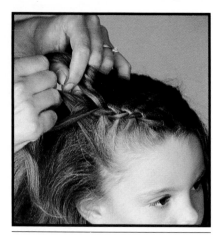

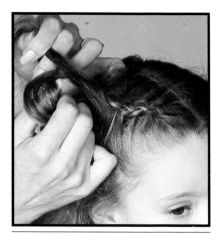

5. Continue underbraiding, but add to the left strand new sections from the area between the hairline and the braid. Add to the right strand new sections from between the part and the braid.

6. As each new, combined strand is formed, reach under the center strand and cross the new strand under it.

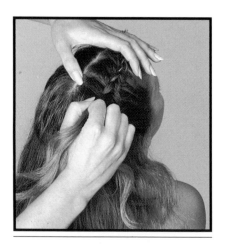

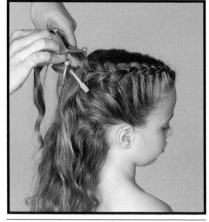

7. As you work toward the back of the head, keep the braid parallel to the center part.

8. When you reach the center back of the head, secure each strand of the braid with clips.

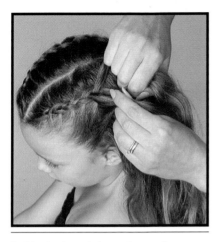 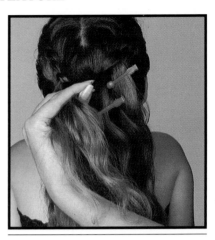

9. Underbraid the other side in the same way, making sure that the positions of the two braids match.

10. When both braids reach the center back, they will be joined together into one braid.

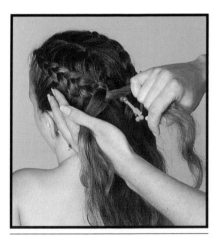 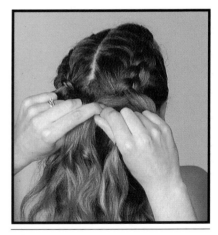

11. Join the center and left strand of the left braid in your left hand. This will be the first strand of the larger braid. Keep the right strand separate.

12. This right strand of the left braid combines with the left strand of the right braid to create a second strand.

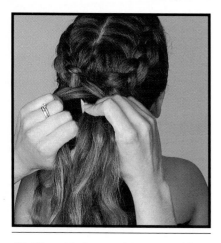

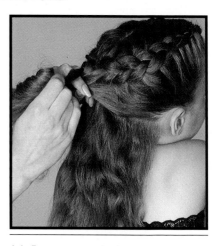

13. The third strand is created by combining the center and right strand of the right braid.

14. Begin to underbraid with the three newly formed strands.

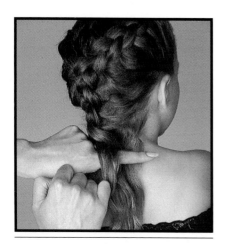

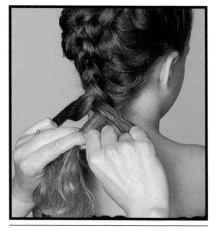

15. As you braid, pick up new sections of hair from either side of the braid and add them to each outside strand.

16. When all of the hair has been picked up from the scalp and added to the strands, underbraid the remaining loose hair.

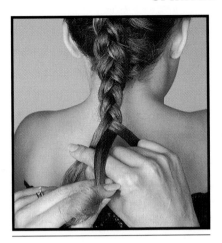 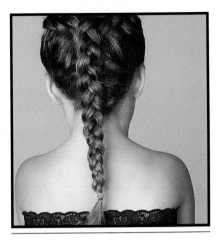

17. Continue to underbraid to the ends.

18. Secure the ends with an elastic band. A barrette or other ornament can be used to cover the elastic band.

CHARMING CONTOURS
ASYMMETRICAL THREE-STRAND BRAID

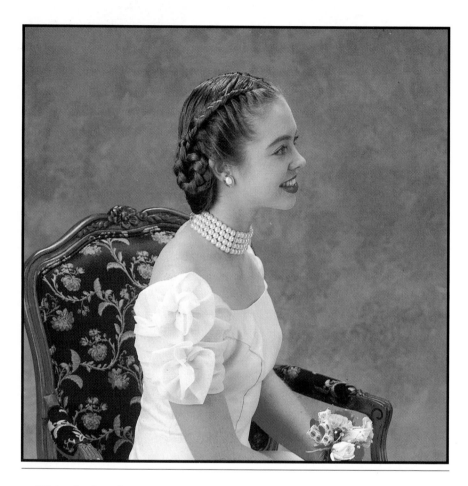

This design is one of the most versatile you'll ever create, as well as one of the most charming. Asymmetrical three-strand braiding makes for intricate patterns and contours framing the face.

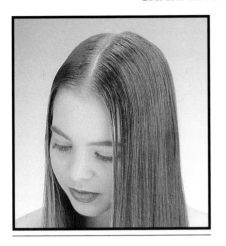

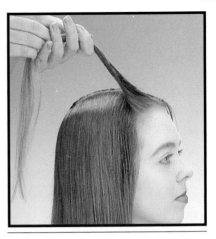

1. Part the hair either down the center or down the side from the front hairline to the nape. Distribute the hair evenly around the head.

2. Part a triangular section at the right front hairline. Direct this section up and back.

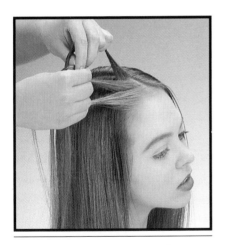

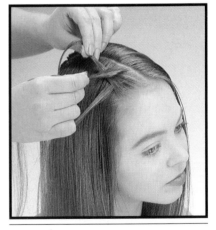

3. Divide the section into three equal-size strands. The strand nearest the hairline is the "outside" strand, while the strand in the middle is "center" and the strand nearest the part is "inside."

4. Begin with the basic three-strand overbraid on the right side of the head. First, cross the outside strand over the center strand. Next, cross the inside strand over the center strand.

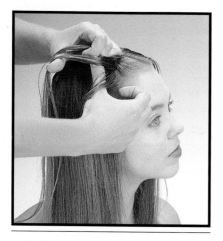

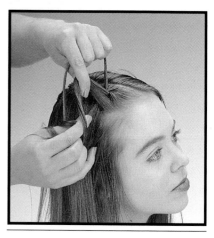

5. Before continuing, pick up a thin section of hair from the hairline area and add it to the outside strand.

6. With thumb and index finger of the left hand, grasp these joined outside strands and cross them over the center strand. Cross the inside strand over the center strand.

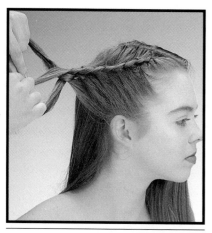

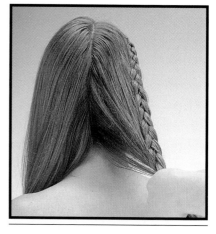

7. Work your way back along a diagonal line, going away from the head. (No additional hair is added to the inside strand before crossing it over the center strand—hair is added only to the outside strand.)

8. Continue picking up strands from the hairline area along clean, diagonal partings. Add these strands to the outside strand until all the hair has been picked up.

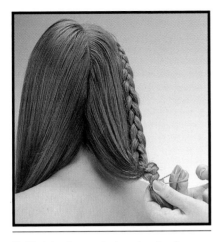

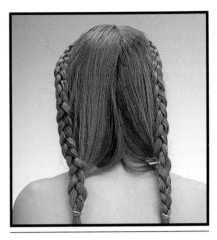

9. Finish the ends in a basic three-strand braid and fasten them with a coated elastic band.

10. Repeat steps 4 through 8 on the left side of the head. Pick up a small strand of hair from along the hairline and add it to the outside strand before crossing over the center strand. Finish the braid and fasten it.

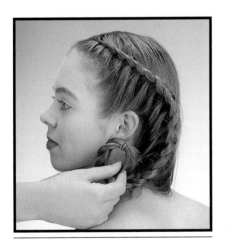

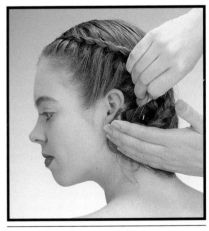

11. Directing the two braids toward the back of the head, roll the ends of each into a bun.

12. Pin in place to secure, and add ornamentation as desired.

VARIATION

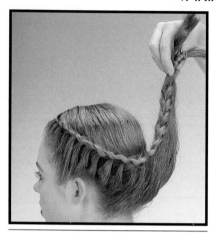 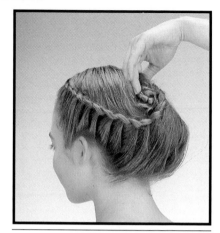

1. Instead of creating two buns, try this variation. Gather the ends of both braids and lift them up toward the crown. Secure the ends together with a coated elastic band.

2. Roll the joined ends under at the crown and pin in place. Then use hairpins to secure both braids to scalp hair. Using this method of pinning relieves tension on the crown. Add decorative accents as desired.

INTRICATE DELIGHT

FOUR-STRAND ROUND BRAID

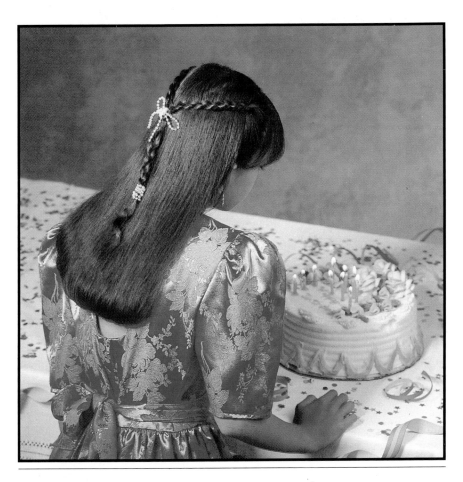

As intricate as this round braid appears, the technique is surprisingly easy. Getting the hang of it is just a matter of synchronizing your hands. You'll soon be on your way to creating many unusual and beautiful designs!

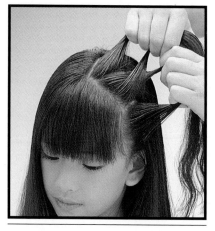

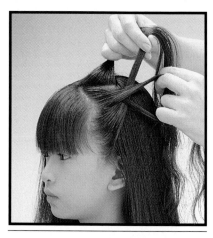

1. Part the hair normally. Section a triangle of hair on one side of the head from the front hairline up to the parting. Divide this section into four equal-size strands. Cross the inside left strand over the inside right strand.

2. With thumb and index finger of the right hand, grasp the outside left strand from behind the two inside strands. Bring the left strand behind the two inside ones . . .

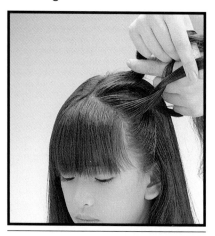

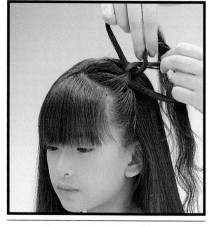

3. . . . and back over the inside right strand. In effect, the outside and inside left strands have switched places. Now, with thumb and index finger of the left hand, grasp the outside right strand from behind the two inside strands . . .

4. . . . and bring the outside right strand behind the two inside ones and back over the inside left strand. Continue this until the braid is long enough to reach the center crown area. Put a clip on the braid temporarily.

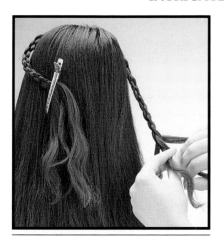

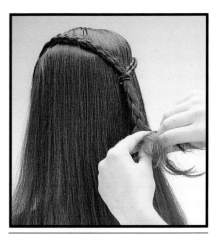

5. Repeat the four-strand braiding technique on the other side of the head. When you reach the center back, unclip the other four-strand braid and fasten the two together with a coated elastic band.

6. Divide the hair that's left into four equal strands. Repeat the four-strand technique described above and fasten the end with a coated elastic band. Add ornamentation as desired.

HIGH SOCIETY

ROLL WITH FOUR-STRAND BRAID

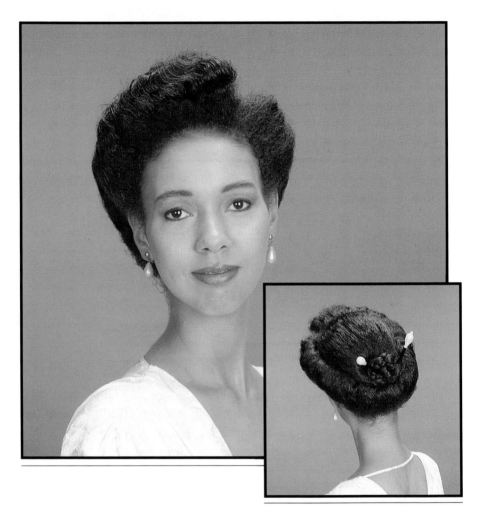

A curved roll around the edges of the hairline sets the foundation for this design. The roll is created by turning smaller segments of hair and pinning them into position to form a curved shape that follows the hairline. Turning the hair segments tightly will produce a smaller roll. An optional accent is the four-strand round braid from the crown of the head.

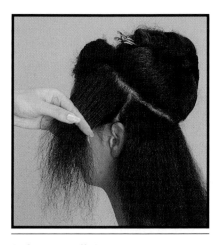

1. Section off the crown in a circular shape and pin it out of the way. Beginning on the side of the part with the least hair, separate a small section and comb the hair smooth.

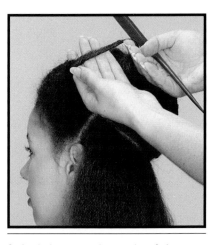

2. Lightly twist the ends of the section so that they form a small strand.

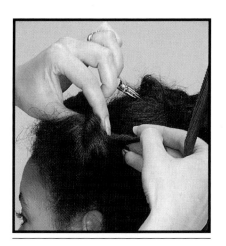

3. Fold the section up and in towards the crown. Adjust the height of the fold so that it is flattering. Tuck the twisted ends inside.

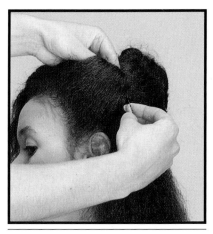

4. Secure the segment with a bobby pin.

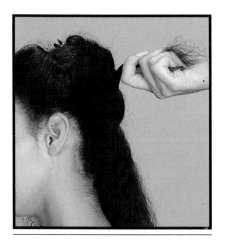 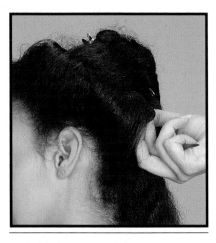

5. Separate the next small segment to continue the roll. The angle at which you hold the hair before you twist is important—check to make sure the new segment will blend with the ones already rolled.

6. Fold the ends of the new segment inside and blend the height to the one already created.

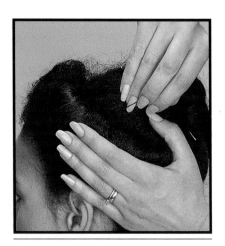 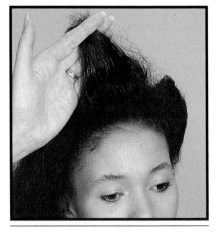

7. Insert hairpins to connect the two segments once the new one is in position.

8. When you have reached the center back, stop and move to the front. Separate a section of hair at the front right next to the first roll that you made.

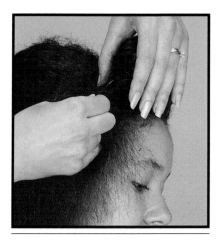 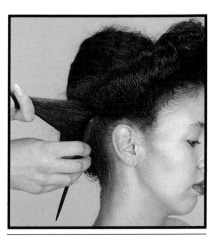

9. Roll the front section carefully to create the desired height. Pin the roll as before. Make sure the height and width of the rolls at the face are flattering. You can then work to blend in that balance with the roll at the back.

10. Work around toward the back, combing each section smooth before directing it upward.

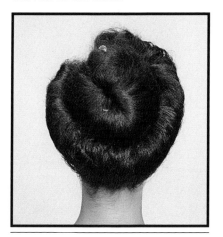 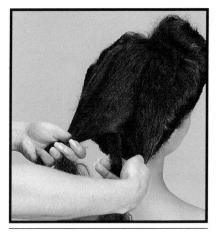

11. When you position the final roll at the back, blend it to the rolls pinned previously. Check to make sure the entire roll is balanced before you proceed to the braid.

12. Release the crown section. Comb the hair back and divide it into four equal-size strands. Cross the two center strands.

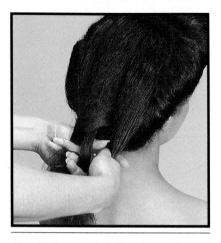

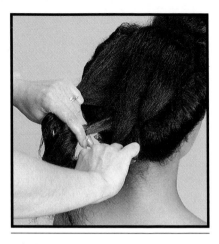

13. With your left hand, reach under to the outside right strand and grasp it.

14. Direct this strand under the two center strands.

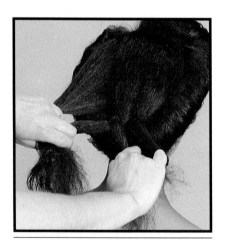

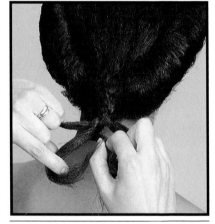

15. Then direct the same strand over the last strand it went under. Repeat with the outside left strand, guiding it under the two center strands and over the last strand it went under.

16. Continue braiding the four strands. Outside strands go *under* two and back *over* one. When you reach the ends, secure them with a coated band.

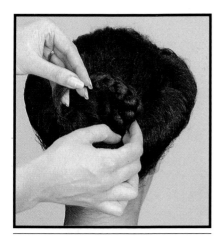 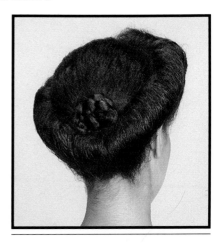

17. Curve the finished braid into a small coil and position it above the rolls of hair.

18. Pin it into place, forming a braided accent to the rolls.

LAVISH DETAIL

TWO-STRAND OVERLAP—FREE

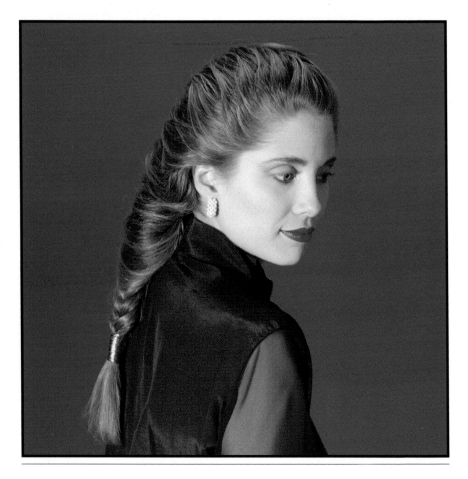

The two-strand overlap produces a herringbone pattern in the hair. It looks like an intricate design, but it's actually easier than braiding with three strands. Working close to the head and keeping tension on the hair will produce a flat pattern. If you work away from the head, the lengths will drape and fall softly around the hairline. The length of the hair will limit how far you can work from the head and still achieve a successful result.

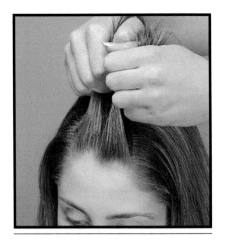

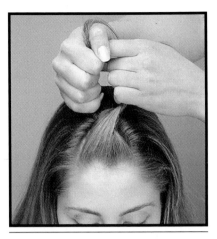

1. Brush through the hair to eliminate all tangles. Section a triangular shape at the front hairline. Divide it into two equal-size strands.

2. Cross these two strands. It doesn't matter if you cross right over left or left over right. Here we crossed left over right.

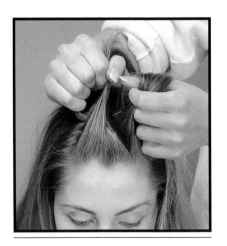

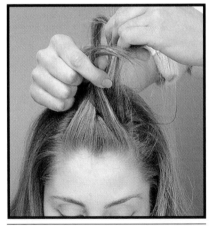

3. Pick up a new section of hair from the right side. Use your thumb to part through from the hairline to the top of the head.

4. Reach across with the thumb and index finger of the left hand to grasp the new section.

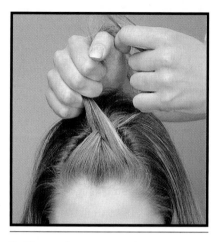

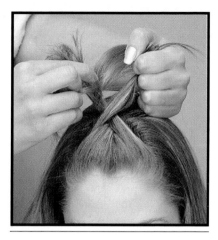

5. Cross the new section over to the left side and join it with the left strand.

6. Pick up a new section of hair on the left side from the hairline to the top of the head. Cross it over and join it with the right strand.

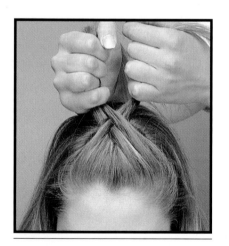

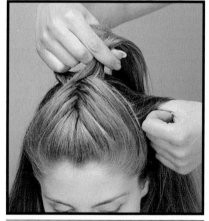

7. Alternate this basic pick-up-and-cross-over pattern. Try to keep the size of the picked-up sections consistent.

8. Hold the two strands in one hand while you use the thumb or index finger of the opposite hand to part through the hair to select the picked-up sections.

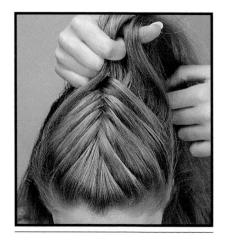 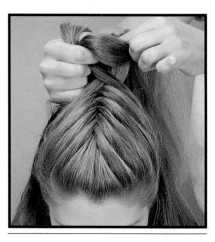

9. Lift the new section upward to the thumb of the hand holding the strands, and then clear away any loose or tangled hair lengths.

10. Grasp the new section and cross it over to the left side. Join it to the left strand.

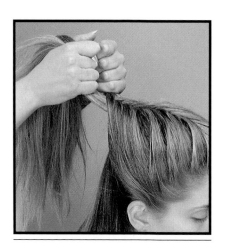 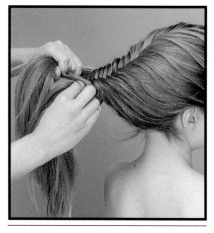

11. Keep your hands close to the head until you reach the crown area. Then allow your hands to move away from the head. This will achieve a draped effect and add fullness to the design.

12. Direct the picked-up sections upward to your hands. Work along an imaginary plane straight back from the head to keep the pattern consistent.

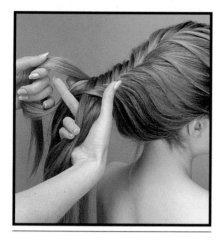

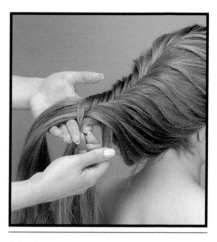

13. After you have picked up all the hair along the hairline, continue the overlap technique on the two strands remaining in your hand. With the two strands in one hand, subdivide a small portion of hair from the left strand.

14. Cross this subdivision over to the right side. Then subdivide a portion of hair from the right side and cross it over to the left. Try to keep these subdivisions equal in size to achieve a consistent pattern.

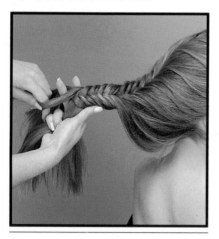

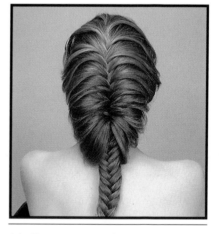

15. Use your fingers to keep the two strands separate as you cross the subdivisions from one side to the other side.

16. Continue overlapping down the length of the hair. Secure the ends with a covered band.

COUTURE

TWO-STRAND OVERLAP—TUCKED UNDER

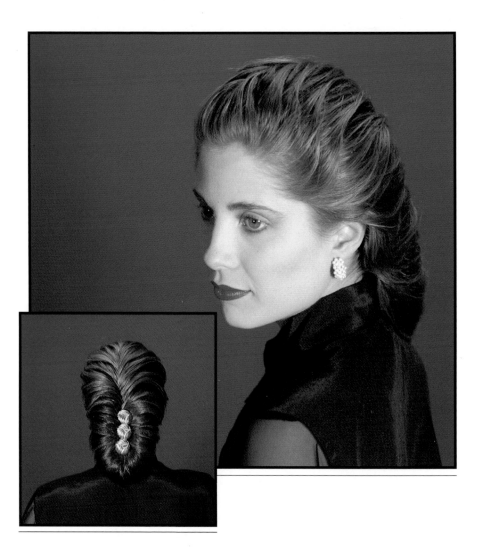

Once a two-strand overlap is completed, you can create a more sophisticated version simply by tucking the tail under and pinning it to itself. For this design, though, you must keep your hands away from the head after you reach the crown so that you achieve enough drape in the hair to enclose the "tail."

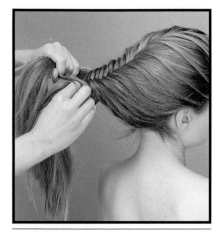

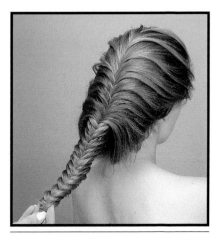

1. Perform a two-strand overlap from the front hairline to the center nape. Notice how far your hands must stay away from the head to achieve a draped effect.

2. Secure the ends with a covered band.

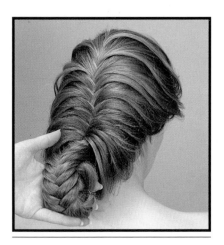

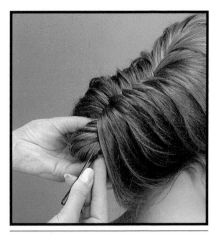

3. Roll the "tail" under and tuck it inside.

4. Pin the roll to itself with bobby pins to secure it in position.

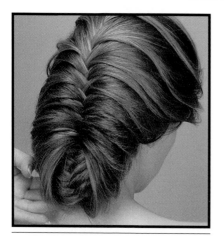

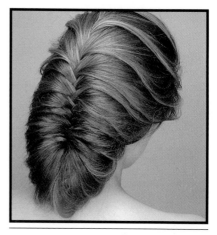

5. The draped lengths will surround the roll.

6. If you wish, you can completely enclose the roll by pinning the edges of the draped lengths together with a hairpin or two.

CAREER MOVES

TWO-STRAND OVERLAP

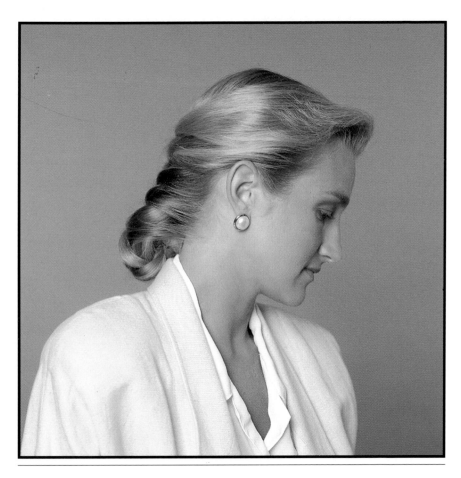

This is a smooth, understated design very suitable for business situations. It requires long hair at the sides. Strands are picked up from the hairline at both sides of the head, brought to the center back, and crossed over each other. A few large strands create a simple look; for a more intricate design, use more strands that are smaller. A draped effect can be achieved by leaving more slack in the hair before pinning the strands in place. In this design, the remaining hair is finished off with a three-strand underbraid.

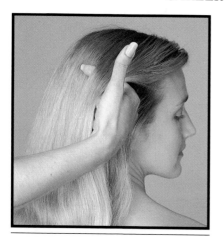

1. Comb the hair smooth and create a side part. Pick up a section from one side of the front hairline.

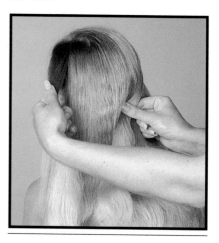

2. Direct the section to the center back. Select an equal amount of hair from the opposite side and direct it to the center back.

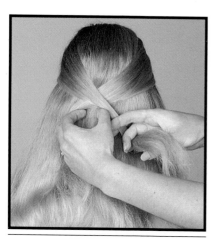

3. Cross the left strand over the right one and hold the two strands in position.

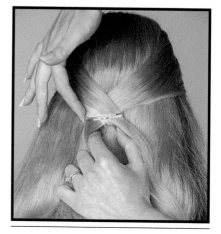

4. Secure the two strands by pinning a bobby pin across the overlap. Position a second bobby pin from the opposite side to ensure a firm hold.

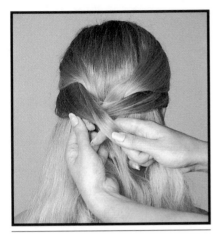

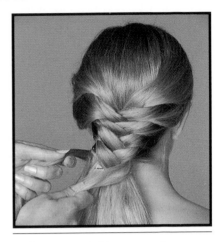

5. Repeat the procedure, picking up, crossing and pinning with two new strands. Position the overlap of the two strands to cover the bobby pins holding the previous overlap.

6. Continue picking up and crossing down the center back until the last section has been picked up from the scalp.

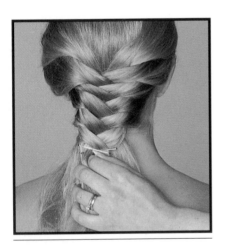

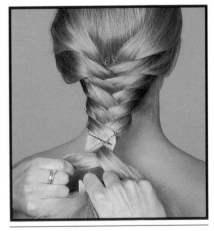

7. Temporarily pin this last crossing to hold it in place. The pins will be removed once the remaining hair is braided.

8. Divide the remaining hair into three equal-size strands. Underbraid by crossing each outside strand under the center strand, alternating from left to right.

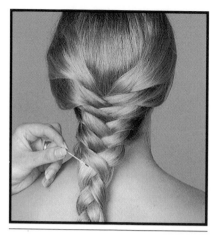

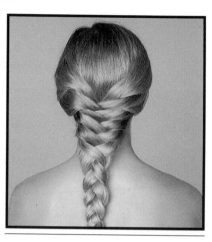

9. Fasten the ends and remove the bobby pins from the last crossing.

10. For a casual look, this design can be worn with the braid hanging free.

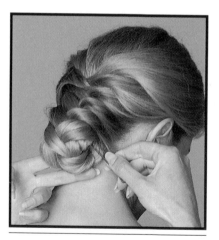

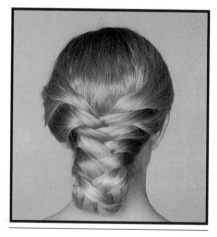

11. To tuck the braid under, curve the end and roll the braid toward the scalp. Secure it underneath by attaching it to the nape of the neck with a bobby pin.

12. Only the two-strand overlap shows in the finished tucked-under version, producing a clean, uncluttered design.

SLEEK AND FESTIVE

TWO-STRAND OVERLAP AND FOUR-STRAND ROUND BRAID

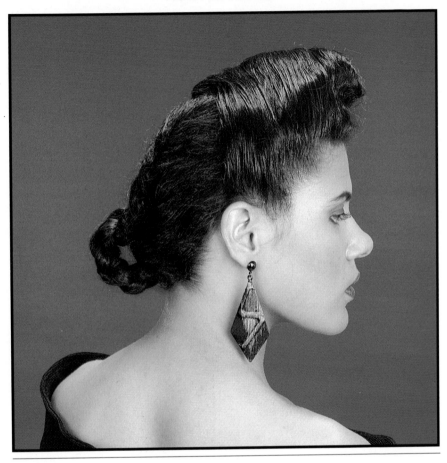

In this glamorous design, each side is done in a two-strand overlap and the two sides are joined in a four-strand round braid. The braid's distinctive chain pattern makes an unusual accent to the smooth look of the top hair.

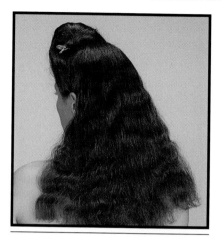

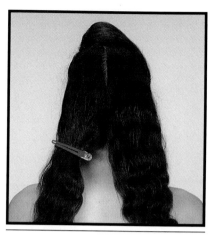

1. Section the front area from the back with a parting that extends across the top of the head from ear to ear. Clip the front area out of your way.

2. Part the remaining hair down the center back of the head. Clip one side to keep it out of the way while you work on the other side.

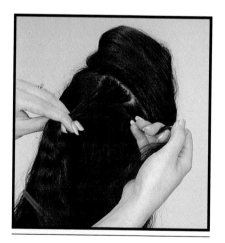

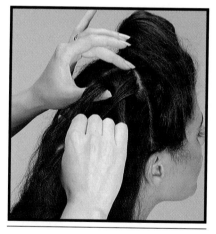

3. Pick up a triangular section of hair at the point where the two parts meet and divide it into two strands. Cross the right strand over the left.

4. Pick up additional hair from the scalp on the left side of the two strands.

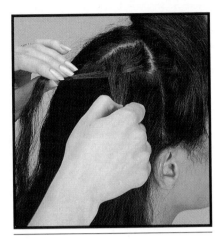

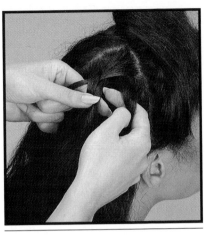

5. Cross this picked-up section over to the right side of the crossed strands and join it with the strand in your right hand.

6. Pick up additional hair from the scalp on the right side.

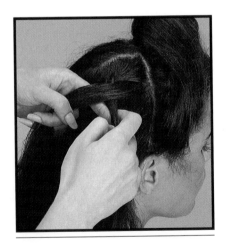

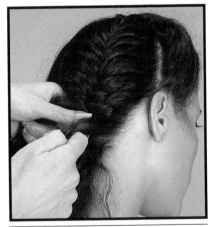

7. Cross this picked-up section over and add it to the strand in your left hand.

8. Repeat this left-over-right and right-over-left overlap down this side of the head.

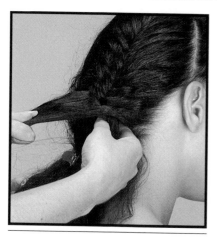

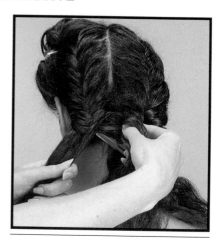

9. Remember to run your hands down the lengths of hair to smooth and untangle the strands before overlapping them.

10. Continue until you have picked up all the hair on the first side. Clip the strands to hold them in place while you repeat the procedure on the other side.

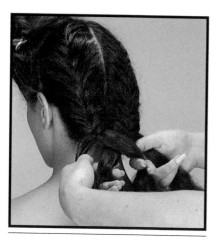

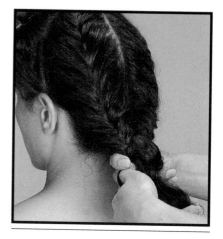

11. You now have four strands—two from each side. You will use these strands to create a four-strand round braid. Begin by crossing the two center strands.

12. Grasp the outside left strand and direct it under the two center strands.

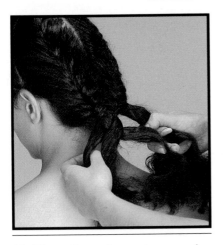

13. Then direct that same strand back *over* the last strand it went under.

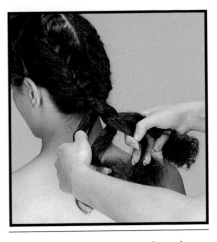

14. Now grasp the outside right strand and move it under the two center strands and back over the last strand it went under.

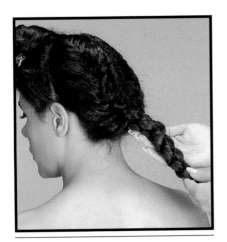

15. Continue braiding the four strands. Outside strands go *under* two and back *over* one. When you reach the ends, secure them with a covered band. Tuck the finished braid under and pin.

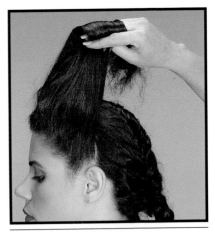

16. Release the top hair and brush it smoothly upward. Hold the ends and fold them under.

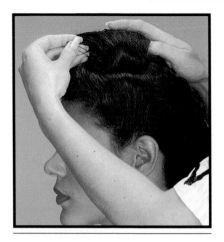 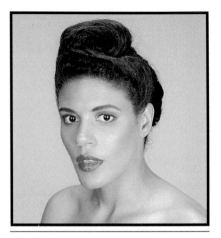

17. Roll the hair down toward the scalp and pin to secure the roll.

18. Make sure the size of the roll balances the total design. Adjust the size of the roll by tucking it tighter or expanding it.

OPULENT

REVERSE OVERLAP WITH DOUBLE ROLLS

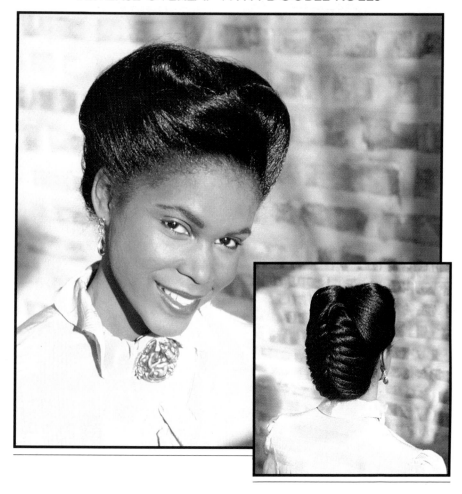

This design uses the overlap technique in a reversed position, working from the nape up toward the crown. It creates a graphic herringbone pattern. You can either work close to the head or, as in this design, slightly away to create an effect with more volume. The number of picked-up sections that you gather will determine the intricacy of the pattern. The rolls in the top front area on either side balance the design in an asymmetrical fashion. You can also use a single roll, as in the style variation on page 97, or if the lengths are shorter, they can be waved or curled.

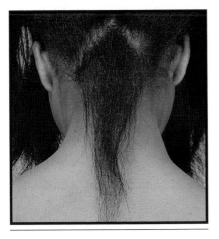

1. Begin at the nape area by releasing a triangular section of hair.

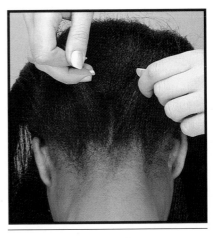

2. Divide this triangular section into two equal-size strands.

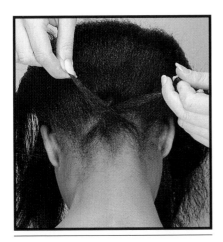

3. Cross one side over the other for the first overlap. Here, the right strand was crossed over the left.

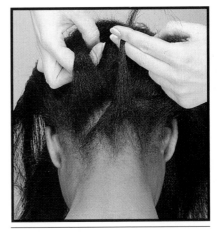

4. Now pick up a new section of hair from the left, sectioning from the hairline to the center back as shown.

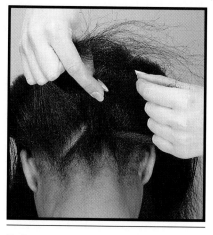

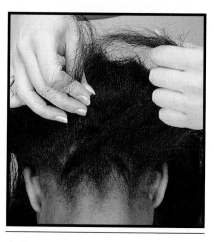

5. Free the thumb and index finger of your right hand so that you can reach over and grasp the new section.

6. Cross this new section over to the right side and join it to the right strand.

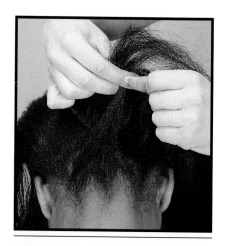

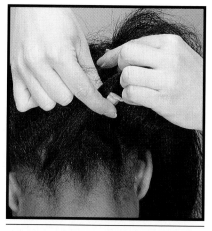

7. Pick up a new section on the right side, sectioning from the hairline to the center back.

8. Reach over and grasp this new section, cross it over, and join it with the left strand.

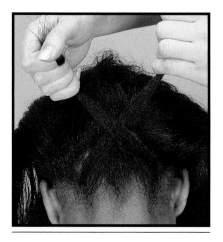

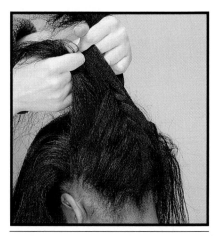

9. Remember that you are always working with two strands in your hands and that the picked-up hair is crossed over and joined with the strand on the opposite side. This creates the overlap pattern.

10. As you work up the back of the head, continue to pick up new sections that extend from the hairline to the center back of the head.

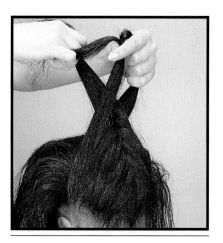

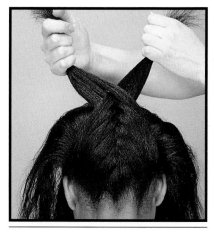

11. Reach over for these picked-up sections and overlap them to the opposite side.

12. The herringbone pattern begins to develop.

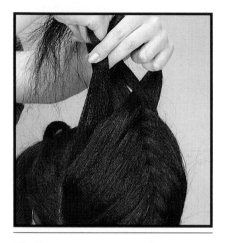

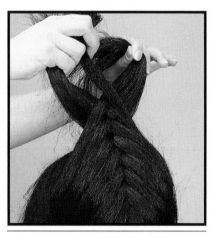

13. If you want extra volume, you can start to move away from the head with the overlap, so that when the overlap is finished it drapes and stands out from the head.

14. Here you can see the final pick-up and overlap in the back area.

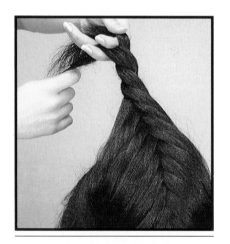

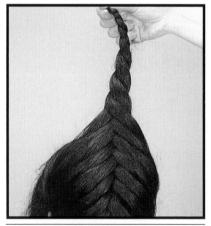

15. Here we've chosen to do a two-strand rope to the ends (see page 100). Note that the index finger is positioned inside the crossover area of the two-strand rope before twisting. This ensures even tension.

16. Work this two-strand roping technique to the ends and fasten.

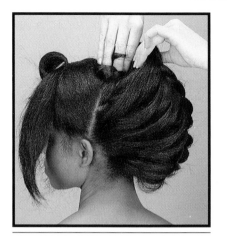

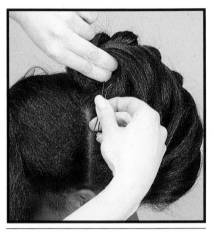

17. The fastened end is circled around and tucked into the gap of the overlap area at the crown.

18. Fasten this topknot with a bobby pin to secure it.

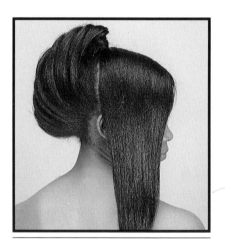

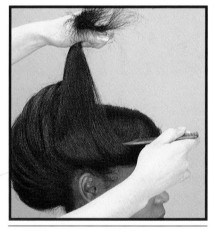

19. To create the rolls, the long hair in the front is parted down the side. Rolls can also be created on shorter hair with lengths of four to six inches.

20. Position a comb at the curve of the head and direct the ends up. This controls the top area and ensures smoothness.

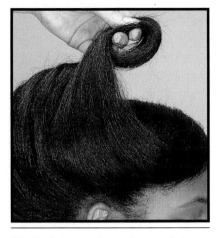

21. Roll the ends under until they reach the scalp area.

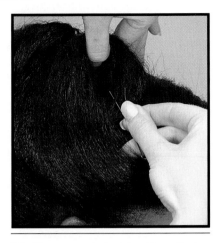

22. Pin securely inside this rolled area with a bobby pin, and insert your fingers to slightly fan the roll outward.

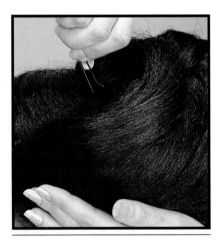

23. Use this same technique on the opposite side.

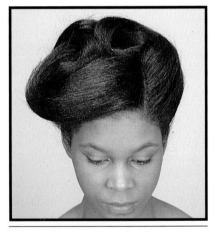

24. We've positioned the double rolls asymmetrically, and they join with the end of the reverse overlap at the crown. You can place the rolls higher or lower, around the hairline, if you wish.

LUXURIOUS

VARIATION: REVERSE OVERLAP WITH SINGLE ROLL

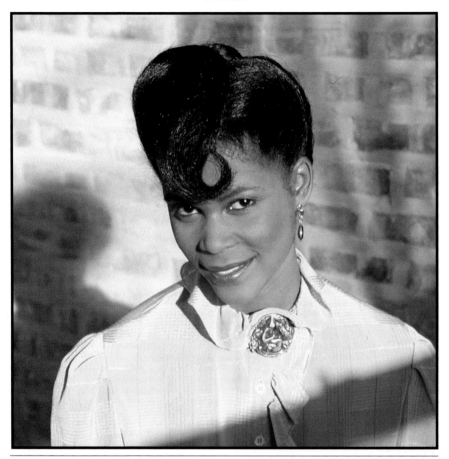

This variation combines the reverse overlap with a single roll. The free ends of the roll create a fringe accent along the forehead. This is a controlled design that is excellent in business situations as well as going out for the evening. The single roll could also be used throughout the entire back area.

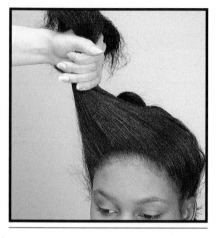

1. The hair is distributed out from the curve of the head as shown.

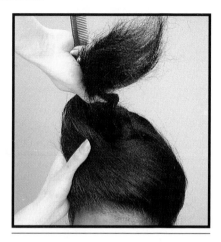

2. Lightly twist the hair ends as you hold the hair with one hand near the base. Begin to direct the twist toward the forehead.

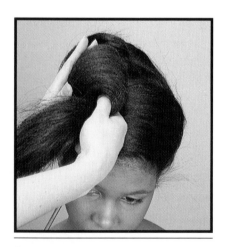

3. Roll the hair with some tension toward the front.

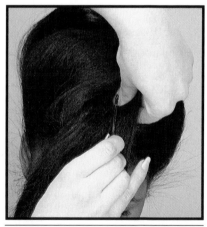

4. Secure inside the roll with a large bobby pin. Add hairpins or bobby pins as needed to secure the roll.

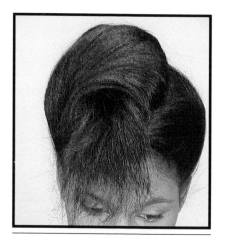 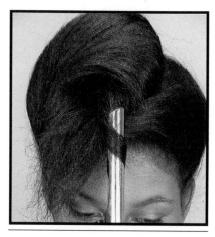

5. The ends are now extending onto the forehead, ready for further styling. They can also be styled straight.

6. Curl the ends as necessary. You can add ornamentation, if you wish.

STREAMLINED

TWO-STRAND ROPE

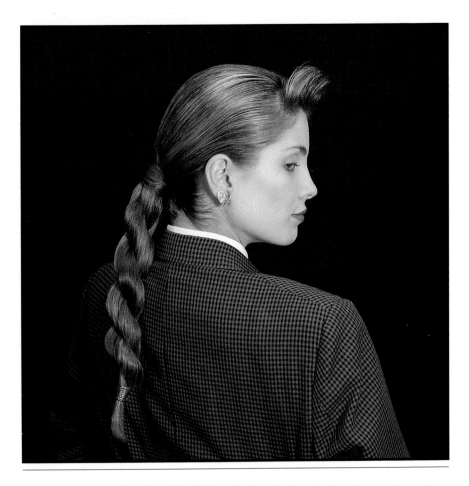

This classic-looking braid variation is based on two strands instead of three. Each strand is independently twisted, and then the two strands are twisted together. This double twist produces a rounded appearance resembling a rope. A successful pattern depends upon remembering to twist the strand that is on top and to twist in one direction only.

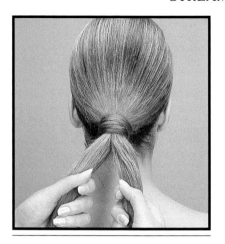

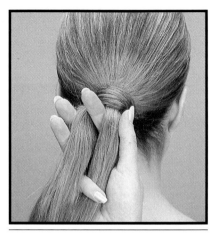

1. Divide the ponytail into two equal-size strands. Slide your hands down the length of the strands to smooth stray ends.

2. Place both strands in one hand, and extend your index finger between the two strands with your palm facing upward.

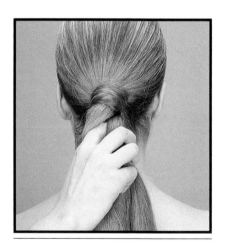

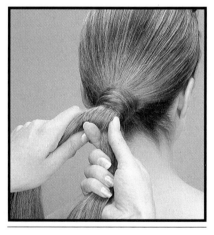

3. Turn your hand over so that your palm faces downward. This will twist the strands, and one strand will be positioned on top.

4. Now twist the top strand toward the center. Hold the strand firmly to maintain the twisted pattern and extend your forefinger between the strands.

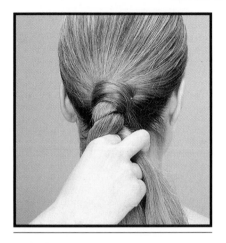

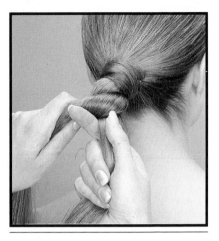

5. Shift the twisted strand to your right hand and turn your hand over, palm down, once again.

6. Twist the top strand, once again remembering to twist toward the center. Extend your forefinger between the two strands.

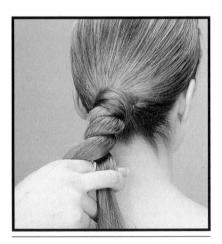

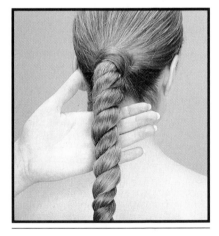

7. Shift the twisted strand so that your right hand holds both strands, and then turn your hand over so that your palm faces downward.

8. Finish the ends by securing them with a covered band or wrapping them with a cord as shown here (see page 9).

YOUNG SPIRIT

ASYMMETRICAL TWO-STRAND ROPE

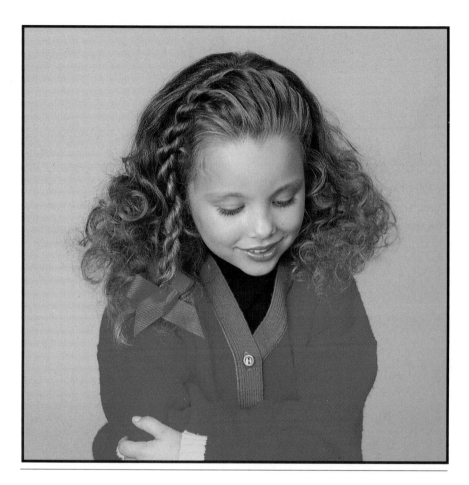

The two-strand rope produces an interesting twisted pattern that is an attractive alternative to braids. When you combine this technique with sections picked up from the scalp, the rope sits on top of the hair the way a projected braid does. The design used here features an asymmetrical rope moving along the front hairline from one side to the other. The hair at the back is left free and can be set with hot rollers for additional curl.

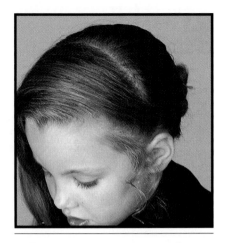

1. Part the hair to separate the front area from the back. Comb the front hair to one side.

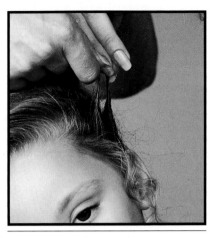

2. Take a rectangular section of hair and divide it into two equal-size strands. Twist each strand clockwise simultaneously. Twist only near the base, keeping your fingers close to the scalp.

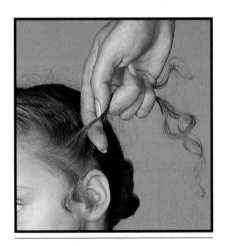

3. Holding your hand palm up, insert your forefinger between the two strands.

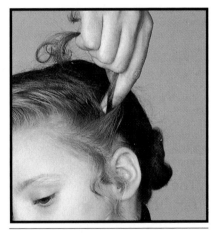

4. Turn your wrist over so your palm is facing down. This automatically twists the two strands together.

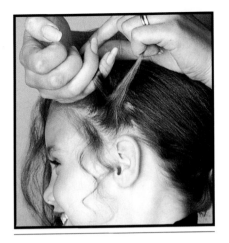

5. Using your little finger, part completely across the front section to pick up a new section.

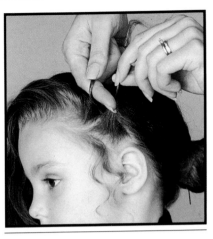

6. Combine the new section with the strand toward the face and twist the combined strand clockwise.

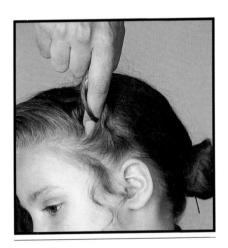

7. Once again, turn your hand palm upward and place your forefinger between the two strands. Turn your hand palm down to twist the two strands together.

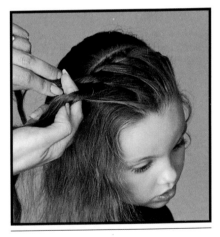

8. Continue creating the rope across the top of the head, adding new sections of hair as you go along.

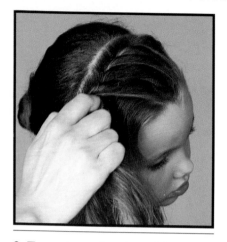

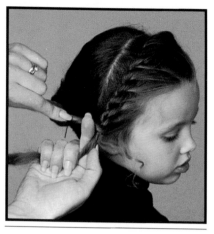

9. Try to keep the size of the picked-up sections equal. This will create an even pattern.

10. Once all the sections of hair have been picked up and incorporated into the rope, continue creating the rope with the remaining loose hair. A turn of the wrist will automatically twist the two strands together.

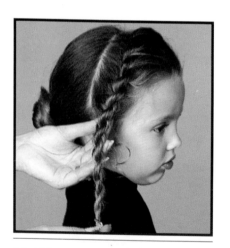

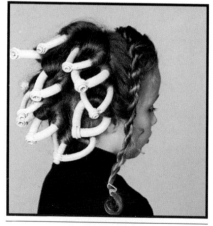

11. When the rope is finished, secure the ends with a coated band.

12. If you want additional curl in the back hair, use a curling iron or spiral hot rollers.

PATTERN PLAY

TWO-STRAND HAIRLINE TWIST

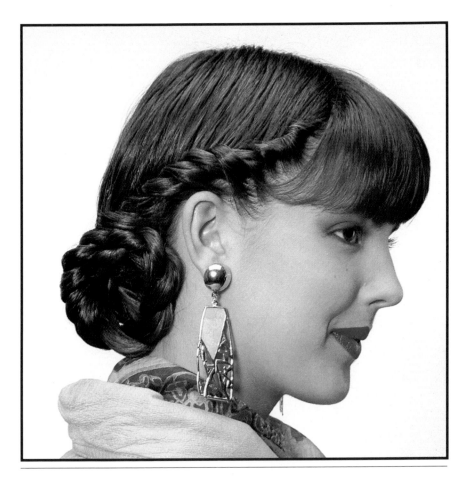

The two-strand twist is a fairly simple technique that involves separating two strands with your index finger and then turning your hand from a palm-up to a palm-down position. This turn of the wrist produces a twisted pattern in the hair. You must remember to reposition your index finger prior to each turn; otherwise the pattern won't be consistent. For this design, you will always be working with two strands, but they will get larger as you gather hair from along the hairline and add it to one side. Keep your hands close to the head to achieve a tightly twisted pattern.

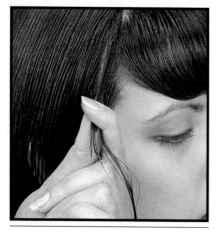

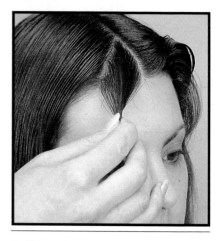

1. Begin by combing the hair as it would fall naturally. Part a small section of hair at the hairline where the pattern is to begin. Here, we started behind the bangs.

2. If you want to incorporate the bangs into the twist, part a triangular section directly off the part.

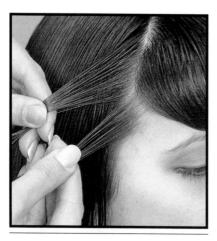

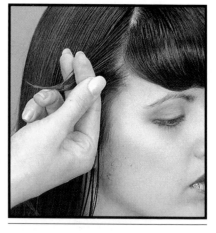

3. Direct the beginning section downward, toward the hairline, and divide it into two strands.

4. Insert your index finger between the two strands with your palm facing upward. Don't forget this step; it is very important to the appearance of the twist.

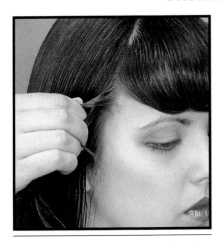

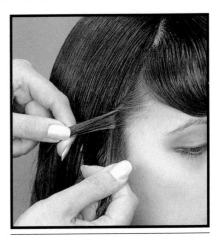

5. Turn your hand over so that the palm is now facing downward. This will automatically position the strands in the twisted pattern.

6. Release the underneath strand and pick up a new section of hair from along the hairline. Combine these together.

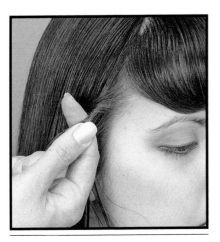

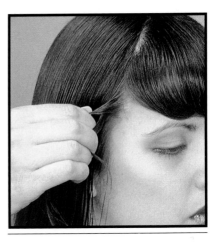

7. Extend your finger between the new combined strand and the top strand.

8. Turn your hand over so that your palm is facing downward.

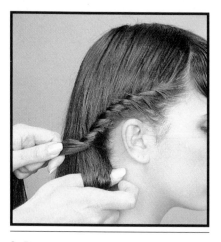

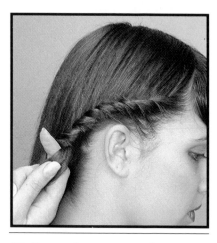

9. Repeat the release, pick-up, and twist steps as you follow along the hairline. Use your thumb and index finger to select the new sections from the remaining hair.

10. Remember to extend your index finger between the two main strands with your palm facing upward.

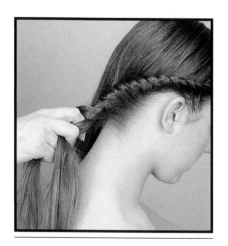

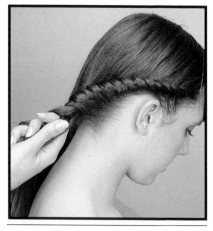

11. Turn your hand over so that your palm is down.

12. Keep your hands close to the hairline and avoid lifting the lengths as you repeat this procedure.

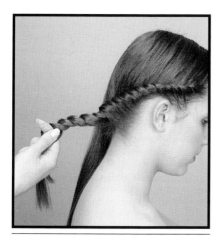

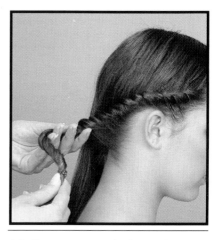

13. Continue picking up hair from the hairline until you reach the center back. Then use the basic two-strand twist technique, without picking up new hair, down the remaining lengths.

14. Once you reach the ends, secure them with a small covered band.

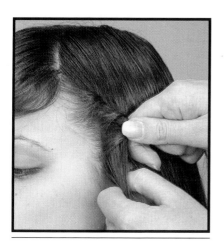

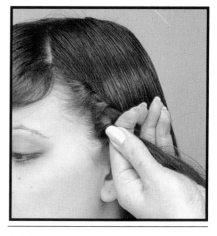

15. Repeat the twisting technique on the opposite side. Follow the hairline once again, and try to match the size of the picked-up sections on this side with the completed side.

16. Remember to position your index finger between the strands with your palm facing upward.

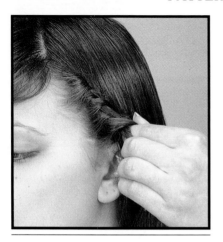 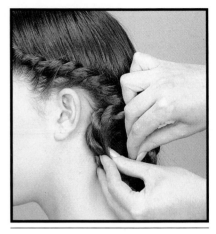

17. Turn your hand over to a palm-down position. Continue around to the center back.

18. When the twist is complete, curve the free ends of the twist into a coil behind the ear. Use a bobby pin to secure it to the head. Coil and pin the twist on the opposite side. Pin the edges of the coils together where they meet.

SHEER FANTASY

SINGLE-STRAND TWIST CHIGNON

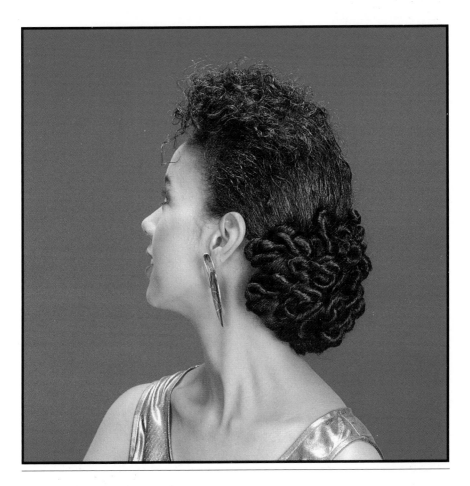

In this design, large individual strands are twisted and pinned in a free-form pattern at the nape. The shape of the chignon can be varied to create an elongated oval in the center back or a wide oval at the nape. Shorter hair lengths around the forehead can be left out to create softness. This design can be created with your own hair, of course, but if your hair is too short you can use an added hairpiece, as we have done here. The first six steps show how to properly attach the hairpiece. The remaining steps show how to create the hairstyle.

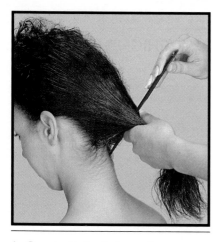

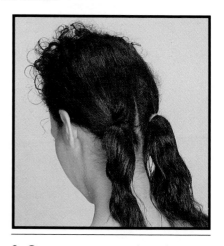

1. Comb all the hair to the center back and divide the hair in half down the middle. A tail comb can help do this quickly.

2. Create two ponytails and secure them with coated bands at the nape.

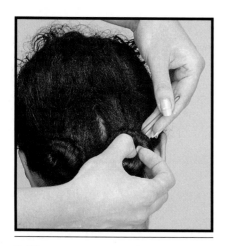

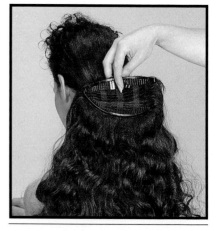

3. Twist one ponytail and wrap it around its base in a coil. Pin it in place. Repeat with the other ponytail.

4. This hairpiece is attached to two combs that interlock when closed.

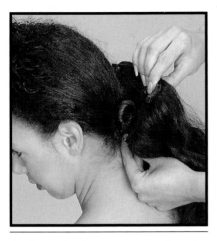

5. Open the hairpiece and place it over the coiled ponytails.

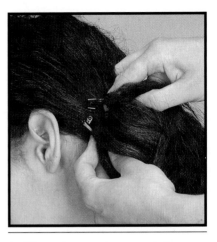

6. Close the comb around the coiled ponytails and snap the ends together.

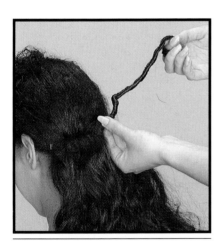

7. Next create the free-form twists. Select a strand from the hairpiece and twist the strand several times.

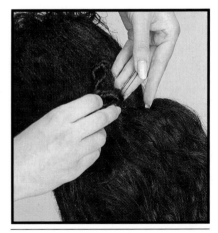

8. Continue twisting until the hair coils and folds. Secure the twist with pins. Work around the perimeter of the hairpiece toward the center.

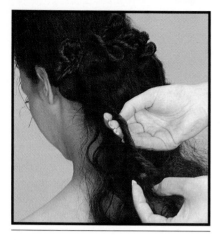

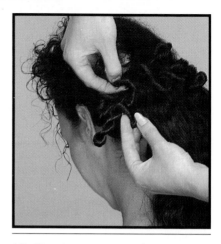

9. Create additional twists and secure them with pins.

10. Continue twisting, being sure to adjust the position of each twist to create a well-balanced design.

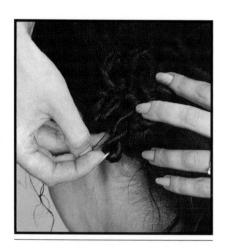

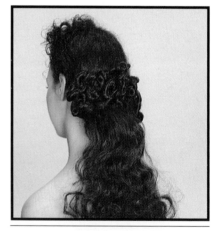

11. Pin each twist at the top and bottom to hold it in position.

12. If you leave some of the hair-piece dangling down, the twisted area acts as a transition between the natural hair and the hairpiece. You can also create twists with the entire hairpiece, giving the hair a more formal look.

MODERN TEXTURE

ASYMMETRICAL CLUSTER OF TWISTS

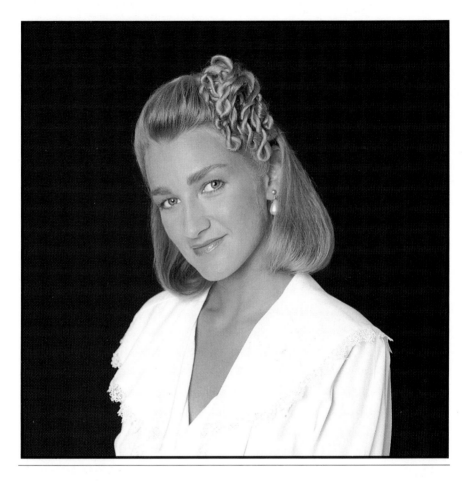

Single-strand twists give a texture completely different from two-strand twists and are very easy to do. Tightly twisting individual strands of hair will force the strands to coil and bend automatically. In this design, several coiled strands are pinned in a cluster on one side of the head, creating a contrast between the smooth pageboy hairstyle and this intriguing texture of twists. This is a free-form technique—the number and size of the twists can vary. Large sections create graphic patterns, and small sections create more delicate twists.

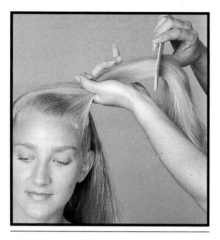

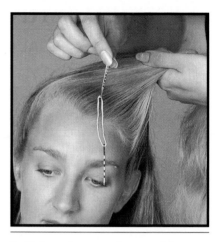

1. Separate a large section of hair at the front and comb it off to one side.

2. Make a fastener by attaching bobby pins to either end of an elastic band.

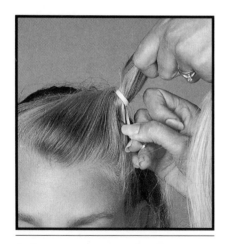

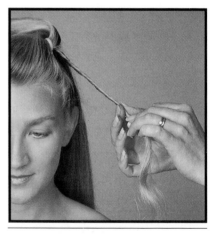

3. Secure the hair at the front in a ponytail by attaching one bobby pin to the base of the hair, winding the elastic band around the hair, and then attaching the other bobby pin.

4. Pick up a small strand of hair from the ponytail. Twist this strand several times.

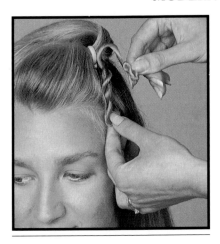

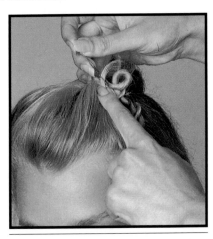

5. Continue twisting the strand until the hair coils and bends automatically. Position the coil against the head so that it suits your design plan.

6. Secure the ends of the twist with a bobby pin. If the hair is very fine, you may need a small bobby pin. Secure the loop of the coils as well. If needed, apply gel to control stray ends.

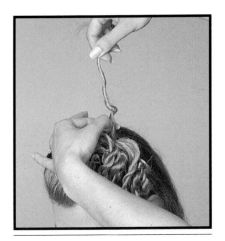

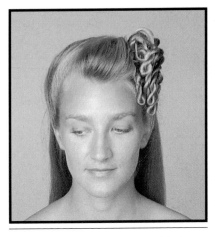

7. Continue to twist and curl the rest of the hair in the ponytail. Keep the size of your twists equal. Check to see that each twist fits in with the design before you pin the top and bottom.

8. The finished twists should show a balanced design with no pins showing.

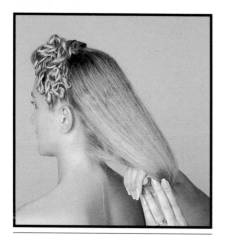 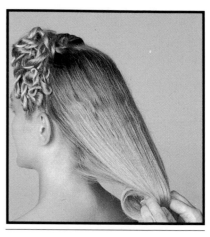

9. To achieve a shorter pageboy look with long hair, roll under several inches of the back hair at the nape. Begin by grasping the ends and folding them back over your hand.

10. Remove your hand and continue to roll the hair up toward the head.

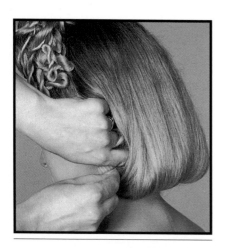 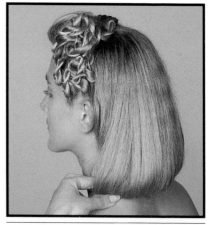

11. Secure the roll by pinning it to the nape area.

12. Finish the pageboy by fanning the edges of the roll behind the ears. This technique offers the option of a shorter look without the permanence of a haircut.

TOP TWIST

SINGLE-STRAND TWISTS

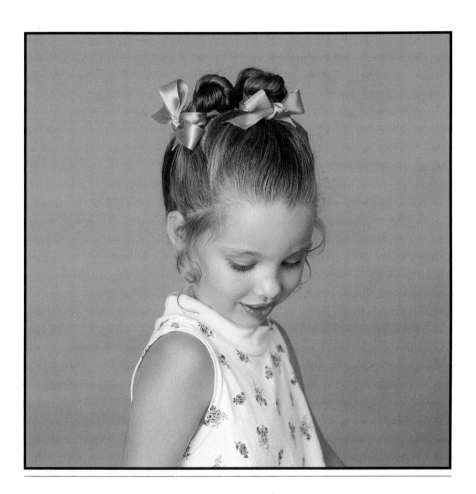

Large twists are fun alternatives to ponytails and a great way to design wet longer hair when something simple and quick is in order. Three twists are placed on top of the head, and each twist is ornamented with a bow tied around its base. Consider this design for a girl straight from the bath or out of the pool. Tip: Conditioner can be applied to the hair first, giving the hair protection for fun in the sun.

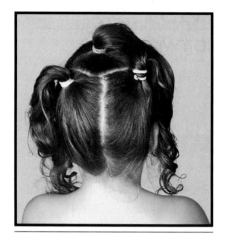

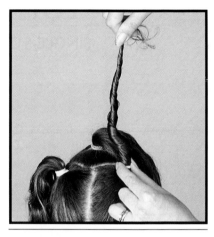

1. Begin by creating three ponytails. Gather the front hair into one ponytail on top of the head. Then divide the back hair in half and create two ponytails behind the center one.

2. Start twisting one of the ponytails. Continue to twist in the same direction until the strand begins to coil and bend over automatically.

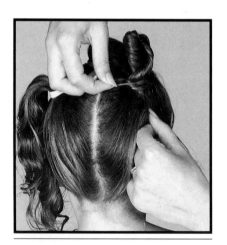

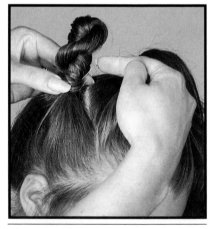

3. Hold the twisted shape in position. Bring the free end down and wrap it around the base of the twist.

4. Insert a hairpin into the base to secure the end.

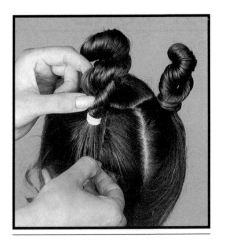 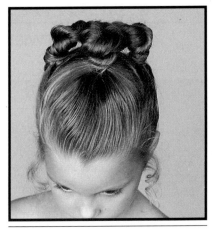

5. Repeat steps 2 through 4 on the other two ponytails.

6. Each twist will take on a character of its own. You can make them stand upright or allow them to fold over. Ribbon can be tied around the base of each twist to dress up the design.

ELEGANT STATURE

TWISTED ROLL

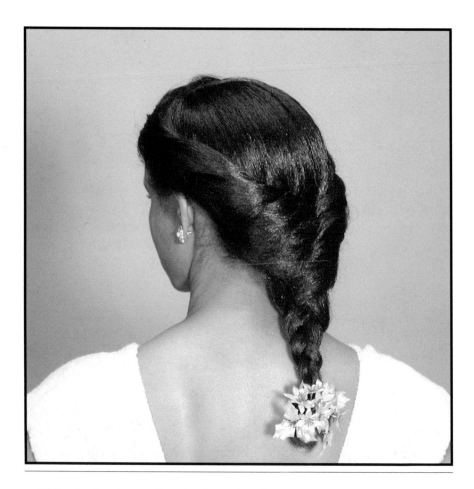

This design is perfect for hair that has some degree of natural texture. You can also add curl to straight hair to give the texture necessary to make this design work well. The twisted rolls along the hairline join together at the nape in a free-falling braid. With shorter hair, the twisted roll can be positioned around the hairline and connected at the center back for one continuous roll. Add a hairpiece at the nape to form into a twist, roll, or chignon. Be creative!

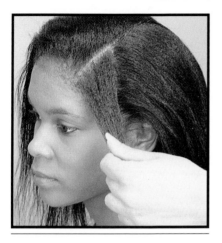

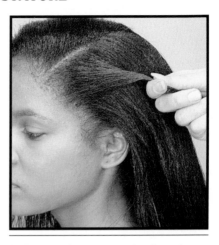

1. Part the hair. Here, a side part was chosen. Define a large triangular section.

2. Direct this section back and away from the hairline. Lightly twist. Don't overtwist; overtwisting will give you a tighter shape with less volume.

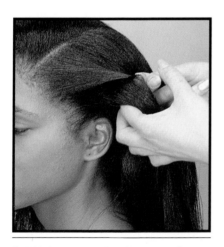

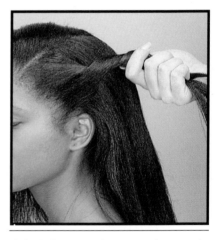

3. With your index finger, pick up a new section from the hairline area. Direct it upward and into your hand. If the hair is long, comb through it with your hand to keep clean, controlled sections.

4. Lightly twist these newly joined sections.

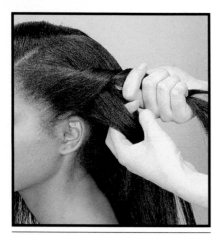

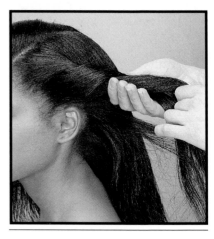

5. Continue picking up hair from along the hairline.

6. Lift it upward and direct it into your other hand.

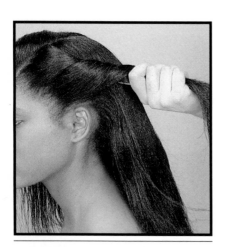

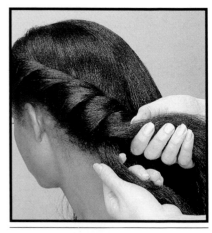

7. Twist lightly.

8. Curve around the hairline area as shown. Note the clear distribution of the hair at the top.

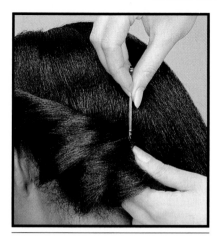

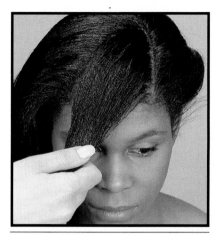

9. Pin the roll with a large bobby pin at the center back before moving to the opposite side to continue with the same procedure.

10. On the opposite side, section a triangular area of bangs. If you prefer loose bangs, pick up your first new section behind the bangs.

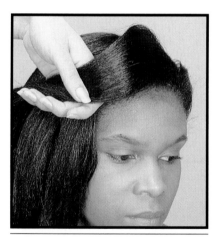

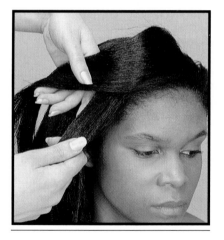

11. Direct this section back along the hairline, letting the hair's natural wave patterns bounce in, if you wish.

12. Continue the twist-and-roll technique. Pick up hair at the hairline.

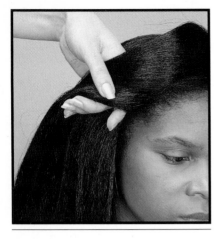

13. Add this new section to the opposite hand.

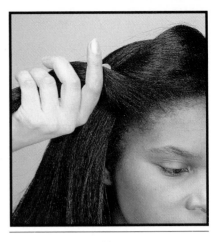

14. Turn the hand to create a twisted roll pattern.

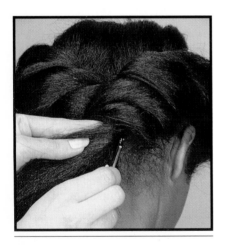

15. Upon reaching the center back, pin the twisted roll in place securely.

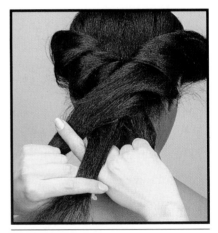

16. These loose ends can be finished off in many ways. We've chosen to underbraid to the ends. Add ornamentation to this design to fit the occasion.